Pregnancy
and Childbirth:
Naturally

Pregnancy and Childbirth: Naturally

Dr Kevan Thorley
and Trish Rouse

BLOOMSBURY

First published in 1997

Bloomsbury Publishing plc
38 Soho Square
London, W1V 5DF

A copy of the CIP entry for this book is available from the British Library

ISBN 0 7475 3021 1

10 9 8 7 6 5 4 3 2 1

Designed by Neysa Moss Design
Typeset by Hewer Text Composition Services, Edinburgh
Printed in Great Britain by Clays Ltd, St Ives plc

FOREWORD

As a mother and busy obstetrician, I was delighted to read this book. The authors, a family doctor and a community midwife, explain clearly how expectant mothers can actively participate in the care they receive before, during and after pregnancy. Encouraging women to ask questions and take informed responsibility for themselves and their baby during pregnancy is a theme which runs from the first to the last page. In the introduction they comment that the 'clinical part of antenatal care should be kept to a minimum and that what is done should be of a high quality'. I welcome this viewpoint with open arms.

The emphasis of this book is on providing clear, sensible and up-to-date information about the options available for antenatal care and childbirth – armed with which the individual woman is able to make informed choices at each step of her journey, from conception to the care of her newborn baby. At each of these stages the authors have drawn upon their practical experience of the needs of their patients and included contributions from a wide range of health care professionals and mothers. As a result, they have created a valuable self-help guide and an enormously practical handbook for mothers, their partners and families during pregnancy.

Their belief that education and support is more important for mothers during the antenatal period than clinical measurements alone is well supported in every chapter. I particularly enjoyed the careful way they introduce the reader to the differences between medical evidence and medical opinion. But the real breath of fresh air comes with the emphasis they place on the importance of randomised controlled trials, evidence-based medical practice and the power of scientific research.

In 'Preparing for Pregnancy' the reader is offered clear guidelines on how to approach pregnancy. In addition to physical considerations, advice is included about the emotional and economical preparations needed to become a parent. Choosing where to have the baby is discussed comprehensively, and although the authors have an impressive track record to offer women who request a home birth, at no time does the advice become directive or biased. For similar reasons the chapter on screening will prove compelling reading for many couples. Screening for abnormality during pregnancy is rarely a black-and-white issue, indeed it is usually grey and cloudy. The importance of individual situations and emotions is strongly emphasised. Most books on the subject of pregnancy and delivery mention the common problems of tiredness, back pain and depression, but this book provides detailed suggestions for recognising these problems and dealing with them.

The final chapter, 'Now What? – The New Baby' is particularly valuable. In addition to checklists of what to ask, what to do and what to buy for the new baby, the authors share with us the experience they have gained from their postnatal clinics. They have identified the fact that experienced mothers are best at providing new mothers with the encouragement they need to breastfeed successfully, and they repeatedly discuss the importance of the mutual support groups they have developed in their practice, which have had an important impact in reducing the feelings of isolation which many new mothers experience.

I would have liked to have had this book beside me when I was pregnant and feel sure that my patients will benefit from it enormously.

Professor Lesley Regan

CONTENTS

INTRODUCTION

*'I felt as if I wanted to know everything
and there wasn't the information there,
even in all the books and everything.'*
Karen, a first-time mother

....

Mothers in pregnancy have a great desire to know what is going on inside them. In previous years, the attitude of professionals caring for them tended to be 'we know best'. Now, due to a revolution in thinking about maternity care influenced by a 1994 Government report called 'Changing Childbirth', women are able to make many more choices about their care. But it is difficult to make choices without the information on which to base decisions. This book has been written for mothers, to help them make their own choices on the basis of information.

We, the authors, are a family doctor and a community midwife working together to provide care to mothers during pregnancy and birth and the early weeks with a new baby. In 1989 we had the radical idea of changing the way we ran our antenatal clinic. We decided to do something quite unheard of – to ask the mothers what we should do. We held a meeting for our current expectant mothers, some mothers who were recently delivered, some colleagues in General Practice and Midwifery and in hospital medicine, and some physiotherapists, osteopaths and other complementary practitioners. The mothers told us what they thought should happen to antenatal care and what were the problems they experienced with the existing system. This resulted in our new system of antenatal care which is based on a weekly meeting between the midwife, family doctor and the mothers.

In the meetings, we discuss aspects of pregnancy, in particular, the concerns of the mothers present. Sometimes we invite guests to lead the discussion: physiotherapists, an osteopath, often an experienced mother. We don't run an appointment system – our mothers can come whenever, indeed as often as they wish, though we do give guidelines about the minimum number of times to come to the clinic and at what stage of pregnancy these visits should happen. Our mothers are encouraged to question the professionals and to share their own experiences and feelings. This usually takes about half an hour but may last up to an hour. Afterwards, there is time for informal discussion over a cup of tea. The midwife and doctor are then available for individual consultation and to perform routine check-ups. We recommend a minimum of five visits to the clinic: at booking, 22, 30, 36 weeks and term. Mothers may consult or have a check-up if they feel the need for it at any other time during their pregnancy. The midwife or doctor may also suggest extra attendances if they consider this necessary for clinical reasons.

We feel that the clinical part of antenatal care should be kept to a minimum but that what is done should be of high quality. We aim to encourage women to take responsibility for themselves and for their births, and to give them the information they need to make choices. They are encouraged to take control of their births in terms of the positions they will adopt, the methods of pain relief they will use and how the birth will be managed. This encouragement is given during the meetings through discussion among the mothers themselves, and with staff and guests.

The physiotherapists and osteopath who visit the clinic regularly help us to show mothers how to minimise back pain in pregnancy and the puerperium. We discuss attention to posture and care in lifting with them. Exercises are taught and treatment is given early for mothers with problems. Recently delivered mothers help to encourage the expectant ones in breast-feeding and care of new babies. An exercise teacher demonstrates safe exercises for pregnancy and we talk about exercise in water and with music. Complementary therapists discuss the use of homoeopathy, reflexology, and aromatherapy in pregnancy. These therapists may make themselves available to the women for consultation after the meeting.

We think that the group is of the greatest importance because of the mutual support mothers can give each other in it. This is of benefit before and after the birth when new mothers can feel very isolated. Recently delivered mothers are encouraged to bring their babies to the antenatal clinic.

The results of this idea have been pleasing because although the caesarean section rate has almost doubled, both in our district and nationally during the time this new clinic has been running, the rate for our mothers has remained at about seven per cent. Our mothers experience fewer problems with perineal tears and episiotomies, more of them have normal births and more breast-feed. We attribute this apparent success to the mothers themselves, acting together as a group which provides mutual support. The group gives our mothers information which empowers them. As part of our research into our method of antenatal care, we interviewed several of our mothers and asked them what they thought about our new clinic. Karen, who gave us the opening quote, was an active participant in the meetings. She was typical of many mothers who feel that pregnancy is a mystery, but one that they desperately want to understand. After all, it is their own body that is involved, and their own baby.

This book may be regarded as the collected wisdom of our meetings with mothers over the last six years. It is based on the things mothers talk about with us, and on their concerns and expectations; on their experience as well as ours.

There is another theme running through the book – that of **evidence**. We believe that the evidence for and against medical and midwifery procedures should be freely available to mothers, and where there is no evidence about such procedures or treatments, mothers should know this. It is not acceptable merely to tell a mother 'we are doing this for the good of your baby'. In our meetings, we try to give mothers the evidence relating to tests and treatments used in pregnancy and discuss it with them. Only in this way can they have the information to make choices about their care.

The word 'evidence' occurs very frequently in this book. When you see the word **evidence** highlighted and/or in a box, it means that the information has been taken from research into a particular subject. This research will usually be in the form of 'Randomised Controlled Trials' (RCT) of a particular treatment or practice. An RCT subjects the treatment under examination to comparison by use of a control group of patients who received either a different treatment, no treatment, or a placebo. It is one of the most powerful scientific tools in medicine, which helps us to decide which treatments are effective and which are not. Fortunately for us and for everyone working in maternity care, information from research in pregnancy has been collected together in the 'Cochrane Database' on computer disk which is updated annually. We have made extensive use of this information in our 'evidence'.

It is often difficult for people to distinguish between **evidence** and **opinion** stated by health professionals. Opinion is usually based on a professional's experience and should not be discounted, but all sorts of biases affect opinions. We recognise that we have our own particular way of doing things and beliefs about how mothers should be cared for. We have therefore tried to show in the book what information we base on *evidence* and what is our *opinion* based on experience but without the backing of research, by highlighting **opinion** in a similar way to evidence.

The book won't answer every question a mother might have, but we hope it will point the way to finding the answer and encourage mothers to keep asking searching questions.

Using the Book

The book is written as a journey from conception to the care of a newborn baby. Each chapter covers a different phase, starting with preparation for pregnancy. At each stage we have provided checklists of things to prepare, people to consult, questions to ask. It should be possible to read the book as a whole, or to use the particular chapter relating to your own stage of pregnancy.

We hope that whether you are a new or experienced mother reading this book, it will help you to make choices about the care you receive in your pregnancy and to feel confident about your decisions.

CHAPTER ONE

PREPARING FOR PREGNANCY

....

A baby has completed its development by about ten weeks after conception, yet, at best, mothers only know they are pregnant for about half of that time. Since this time of development is crucial (all the baby does after that is grow!) it follows that preparation for pregnancy is very important. However, little attention seems to be given to this by health workers or by prospective parents. There is an increasing feeling that preparation for pregnancy, or 'preconceptual care', can help to ensure healthy babies. We think that preparation should involve the whole person, in their physical, psychological and spiritual aspects. Putting it simply, it makes sense to be at your best physically and emotionally before conception.

When to be pregnant

If prospective mothers and fathers are able to prepare for pregnancy, then part of the preparation may involve timing. Thankfully, even in the technological nineties, we're not yet able to decide precisely when we will conceive. Many pregnancies are unplanned and many happy healthy families result from these 'accidents'. We couldn't pretend to advise about when a couple should plan to have a baby, but here are some points to consider and discuss together:

- **Age** – how old would we like to be when our children are growing up?
    - for older mothers, the risk of fetal abnormalities increases (see Chapter Four)

- are we old enough to have sufficient experience of life to cope with children?
- **Accommodation** – have we got somewhere for a child to live? Babies don't need much room for the first year, but as they grow, more space may be desirable.
- **Existing children** – what sort of a gap in age would we like? Closeness has its advantages – the children may be playmates and friends – but a larger gap may also work, with the older children helping to care for the younger ones to their mutual benefit.
- **Finance** – babies can cost very little for the first few years, but their needs increase as they grow.
  - if mother or father has to give up work there will be a financial cost.

HOW TO BE FIT FOR PREGNANCY

Physical Fitness

Regular exercise is known to improve health, both physical and psychological. It makes you feel good, look good and may help to prevent illness. You don't need to do strenuous exercise for health. Anything which you enjoy and can do regularly (twice a week) for about half an hour and which will increase your heart rate by about ten beats per minute is good. Gentle exercise can be continued in pregnancy: exercise in water, which may or may not involve swimming, has been shown to be particularly beneficial. If you don't like water, then play badminton or tennis, walk briskly, cycle or go to an exercise class. There are many other ways of keeping fit and most forms of exercise are safe in pregnancy, but if in doubt, consult your midwife or doctor.

Healthy Eating

There's no special diet for preparing for pregnancy, but it makes sense that to be at our best, we should eat healthily. It is generally agreed that a good diet should contain:

- *fresh fruit and vegetables* which contain *vitamins* and *fibre*. Raw or lightly cooked fruit and vegetables contain more of these good things;

- *cereal foods* such as potatoes, pasta and wholemeal bread, which are another good source of fibre;
- *protein* which is found in meat, fish, poultry, eggs, cheese, beans, peas and nuts;
- *calcium* which is found in dairy products such as milk, cheese and yoghurt. Calcium is needed for growing bones but has also been found to prevent high blood pressure in pregnancy. An adult woman needs about 1 gram of calcium per day. Three quarters of this amount (750mg) can be found in a pint of milk. An average size pot of yoghurt contains 150mg and cheese is also a good source. A good amount of calcium in the diet also helps to prevent softening of the bones (osteoporosis) which affects many women in old age;
- *folic acid* which is a vitamin known to be vital for development of the baby. It is found in green leaves – cabbage, spinach, lettuce, broccoli and sprouts, and in peanuts. It is needed for development of the baby's spinal cord.

FOLIC ACID

Evidence There is good evidence that taking folic acid before pregnancy helps to prevent abnormalities of the spinal cord and nervous system, like spina bifida. The recommended dose is 4mg per day as a supplement to the average daily intake from fruit and vegetables of about 2mg per day.

Women who have had a baby with spina bifida have an increased risk of carrying a baby with this condition again. Research has shown that taking a folic acid supplement before pregnancy reduces this risk by two thirds. The dose needed for women who have already had an affected baby is 5mg per day, starting before pregnancy and continuing for the first three months.

Multivitamins

A Hungarian research study has shown that congenital abnormalities other than spina bifida, including heart defects, were prevented by taking multivitamins before pregnancy and in early pregnancy. This research needs to be confirmed, but it is safe to take multivitamins, and prospective mothers may feel that this would help their own fitness before pregnancy. The multivitamins should contain at least vitamin C, vitamin B12, vitamin B6 and zinc, in addition to folic acid.

Minerals – good or bad?

Our bodies need various 'trace elements' – mainly metals such as zinc, potassium and magnesium – in tiny amounts in order to function properly. Some experts in nutrition argue that these elements are important in pregnancy and that deficiency of minerals in our diet may in some way be related to problems with conception and to abnormalities in the baby. Foresight, a charity devoted to promoting 'preconceptual care', emphasises the importance of these elements as well as other aspects of the environment, which may influence fetal growth and development, such as food additives and pesticides. They argue, with good logic, that by maximising the health of parents before conception, it may be possible to improve the outcome of pregnancy. At present, however, there is not enough evidence from research to be sure which, if any, minerals are important, and which environmental hazards should be avoided. We know, for example, that high levels of lead found in industrial workers can reduce fertility and that the intelligence of children who have high levels of lead in their blood is lower, on average, than that of children with normal levels. Avoiding all potential toxic substances and taking mineral supplements can result in a rather problematic lifestyle, but for those who wish to try this council of perfection, contact Foresight (see **Addresses**).

SMOKING

Evidence Smoking is known to cause low birthweight (see also Chapter Two) and logically, it would be best to give up before becoming pregnant, not only because of any possible effect on the baby at conception but also because it's probably easier to stop beforehand. Smoking in pregnancy increases the risk of miscarriage by 25%, the risk of stillbirth and neonatal death by 30%, and the risk of premature labour twofold. On average, babies of women who smoke weigh 200g less than the babies of non-smokers. There is also an increase in the risk of antepartum haemorrhage (bleeding before the birth). Babies whose mothers smoke during pregnancy are more prone to chest disease in the first year of their lives, and there is a twofold to threefold increase in the risk of cot death.

ALCOHOL

Evidence Research by the Medical Research Council showed that for mothers who drank any amount of alcohol – even the occasional drink – during pregnancy, their babies' birthweights were lower and there was a higher incidence of abnormalities. Therefore, the best advice is don't drink at all when you are pregnant. It would be logical to extend this to preparing for pregnancy too – say for three months before conception. However, other research seemed to show that an occasional drink did not affect the outcome of pregnancy (see also Chapter Two), so mothers who have the odd lapse should not feel guilty!

Opinion We still feel that the best advice is don't drink when preparing for pregnancy.

Medicines and Drugs

We'll use 'medicines' to describe pharmaceuticals prescribed by doctors or bought over the counter, and 'drugs' to describe drugs of abuse. Some medicines are known to be harmful to babies. Others are known to be safe but for most there is uncertainty, so again the best advice is if there is any doubt about taking medicines, don't. For some conditions which need control by medicines though, we have to balance the potential risk to the baby against the risk to the mother of not taking the medicine. Epilepsy is a common example of such a condition which we'll discuss in detail in the next section.

High blood pressure (hypertension)

This needs to be kept under control during pregnancy, but some of the drugs used to control blood pressure are dangerous to the baby and should be stopped before becoming pregnant. These drugs are known as ACE inhibitors. They may cause oligohydramnios (too little fluid around the baby), or may damage the baby's kidneys. If you are taking one of these drugs, you should consult your doctor before becoming pregnant about changing over to some other treatment to control blood pressure. The ACE inhibitors have names which usually end in '-pril'; examples are captopril, enalapril, lisinopril and perindopril. Most other drugs for high blood pressure are probably safe to take, but there is some doubt about the safety of beta-blockers as they may inhibit the growth of the baby. Examples of beta-blockers are propranolol, atenolol and metoprolol; there are many others, their names usually ending with '-olol'.

There is some evidence that low-dose Aspirin may help to prevent pre-eclampsia (high blood pressure with complications), but the research is not yet conclusive.

It's best to avoid taking over the counter medicines, even aspirin and paracetamol, when preparing for pregnancy, but again compromise may be necessary if, for example, you have a bad headache.

Drugs and solvents are definitely harmful to babies and should be stopped if you are planning to become pregnant. Seek help from your doctor or local Druglink.

How do drugs (medicinal or non-medicinal) affect the baby?

In the first two weeks after conception, the egg travels down the fallopian tube to the uterus where it becomes implanted six to seven days after conception. While this is going on, the cells in the egg are dividing rapidly so that by the second week a cluster of cells has formed the embryo. *Teratogenic* drugs (drugs which cause fetal abnormalities) or, indeed, other chemicals taken at this stage probably have an 'all or nothing' effect. Damage to most of the cells probably causes the death of the embryo before the woman knows she might have been pregnant; therefore, drugs taken during this period may contribute to apparent failure to conceive.

From three weeks on, the embryo begins to develop into three layers of cells from which all the organs develop. Some organs develop earlier than others – the central nervous system, including the brain, develops before the face and kidneys. Drugs taken at this stage – from three to eight weeks – have the greatest potential to cause damage to the baby by interfering with the process of organ development. Little is known for certain about which drugs can cause harm. Vitamin A analogues (isotretinoin and acitrecin) are known to damage the nervous system and cause severe physical and mental defects, but many other drugs may be harmful too.

Since most of this crucial time of development is before a woman could possibly know she was pregnant, it is best to avoid all medicines if possible when preparing for a pregnancy.

Medical Problems

Epilepsy

Most people with epilepsy now lead normal lives and more women with epilepsy are choosing to have children. In the UK there are about 75,000 women with epilepsy who could have children. One pregnancy in 200 occurs in a woman with epilepsy.

The danger of having fits which may in themselves cause injury to the baby outweighs any small risk from the medication itself (see Chapter Six). Changing over from one anticonvulsant to another can result in a fit, which will at the least affect the issue or continuation of your driving license, so this needs to be carefully weighed and discussed with your doctor. Most experts recommend that, if possible, patients with epilepsy should change, before becoming pregnant, to the safest anticonvulsant at the lowest possible dose, and to treatment with one drug only if they are taking two or more. If you have epilepsy, but have not had a fit for a year and are willing to take the risk of fits returning, then it may be best to stop anticonvulsant treatment **under medical supervision** before conceiving and up to the end of the first three months of pregnancy. This will reduce significantly the risk of congenital abnormality in your baby. The risk of recurrence of fits is about 25% by nine months and 40% by two years after stopping treatment. If in doubt about your medication consult your doctor.

There appears to be little to choose from in terms of safety between the three most commonly used anticonvulsants. Women taking anticonvulsants should certainly take folic acid before becoming pregnant.

The risk of a child of an epileptic mother developing epilepsy is higher than for children of women who do not have epilepsy. For women with partial seizures, the risk is 3% but for those with generalised fits it is 5% to 10%.

Diabetes

This is also a common chronic disease which can affect both mother and baby. Unfortunately for the diabetic mother, there is an increase in risk of congenital abnormalities up to three times as great as for the children of non-diabetic mothers. Research shows that improving diabetic control **before** pregnancy can reduce this risk substantially, so for diabetic women planning to become pregnant, the best advice is to pay very close attention to your diet and to whatever treatment you may be using, and to monitor your blood sugar and urine very carefully in the months before you plan to conceive. Seek the help of your doctor or local diabetic clinic if necessary. The good news for diabetics is that there is no evidence of any long-term ill effects from their diabetes on the development or intelligence of their children.

Infection and Immunisation

Some infections of the vagina and cervix are known to cause miscarriage. It is possible that these may remain unrecognised. Chlamydia is a bacterium which causes discharge but sometimes produces no symp-toms. It's a good idea to go for a cervical smear, either at your GP's surgery or at your local clinic, when planning a pregnancy. Infection may be noticed during the examination. If you think you're especially at risk of infection either because you have symptoms – vaginal discharge or pain with intercourse – go to your doctor and ask for swabs to be taken from your cervix to check for chlamydia or other infections. Clearing these up before getting pregnant is important.

Most people know that German measles (rubella) can have a disastrous effect on the baby. What many don't know, however, is that the protection you got when you were immunised as a child can wear off. We recommend that every woman planning a pregnancy should have her immunity to rubella checked before conception. Just ask your GP for a blood test for rubella antibodies.

Work

This is an important influence on the health of workers but there is little evidence of the effect of work on pregnancy and fertility. Two types of hazard at work should be taken seriously: toxic chemicals and radiation. These days most toxic chemicals used at work are subject to strict control and it is the employer's duty in law to inform the workforce of the hazards and to provide proper protection.

People working with lead are especially at risk from problems associated with pregnancy and fertility. Exposure to lead in pregnancy can cause miscarriage, premature labour and stillbirth. Pregnant women should not, by law, be exposed to lead. Industries where lead is used include the manufacture of batteries, paints and rubber products, and glass. Many women work in these industries.

Hospital workers exposed to anaesthetic gases are also at risk of problems with pregnancy and fertility.

Despite the controls and the law, people are still often exposed to toxic chemicals in the workplace.

June consulted us because of problems with infertility. She had been investigated extensively by specialists. When we enquired closely about her life, we found that she was self-employed in her own furniture-stripping business. She was using toluene, a highly toxic chemical, without adequate protection.

Radiation can also affect pregnancy and fertility. This applies mainly to hospital workers who may be exposed to X-rays or other radiation in radiotherapy units. There is, however, a source of radiation which is much more common, the effects of which are controversial, and that is the VDU or computer screen.

RADIATION AND THE VDU

The **evidence** at present is confusing, but is mainly reassuring that VDUs are safe. Some studies, however, have shown an increase in the miscarriage rate for women working at VDUs. Because of the conflicting evidence, the Health and Safety Executive has prescribed limits to the time which women of childbearing age and women in early pregnancy may spend working without a break at VDUs.

Age

Statistically, the risk to a baby born to a woman over the age of 30 is greater than that for a woman under 30. However, there are various factors which influence the statistics which are not physiological. One of the most important is that the risk of Downs' syndrome increases from approximately one in 2000 births at age 20, to one in 109 births at age 40. We'll discuss screening for Downs' syndrome in Chapter Four. Many other social and nutritional factors which apply to pregnancies in older women are probably more important than the age itself. Nevertheless, doctors tend to classify women over 35 as 'higher risk', and women over 35 having a first baby as '*elderly primigravidae*'.

AGE

Opinion We think that most women over 35 are fit and healthy, especially if they get a good diet, don't smoke and take regular exercise. Women in this age group are, in fact, more likely to be fit on these criteria than younger women.

Evidence There is no evidence that these women have longer or more difficult labours, or labours with a greater risk of complications than younger women. Given appropriate screening for the baby, there should be no problems for you if you are placed in this more mature group.

Fitness for Fathers

Little research has been done on the effect of the health of fathers on babies, and little attention is given to fathers' health before pregnancy, but since half the baby's genetic make-up comes from the father, it is likely that the same principles apply to the father's health as to the mother's. Although there is no evidence for this, it makes sense that fathers too should be at their peak of physical fitness (at least to get ready for the sleepless nights when the baby arrives!) and that they too should have a good diet and avoid excessive alcohol and smoking before conception. Most GPs will be delighted to give potential fathers a check-up (in fact, this can usually be done by a Practice Nurse) but very few seem to take advantage of this service.

Mind and Spirit

There is no doubt that having a first baby is the biggest change in any person's life. Most of us found that nothing prepared us for this change. Be aware of it though. Your life (or lives) will never be the same again. There is a small, weak new person coming into your life who will depend on you totally for everything – and this is going to last for 16, 20 years and probably more! Perhaps if you're not sure at this stage about preparing for a pregnancy, the best advice is don't! Not everyone has the luxury of being able to pick the best time in their lives for a pregnancy and for some there never will be a 'best time'. For couples, it's a good idea to talk these things over beforehand, then at least you can help each other to prepare.

The pregnancy itself may bring changes even before the baby is born; mothers tend to feel strongly about their babies and fathers may begin to feel isolated. Strong emotions begin to develop with every change in the baby inside – the first awareness of a 'bump', the first stirrings of movement. When a first baby comes along there will inevitably be a change in a couple's relationship; previously one-to-one, it now becomes triangular. Further changes in the family result from the introduction of second and more babies. Support from friends and family through these changes is very important for both parents. Professional help is always available when there is no 'network' of friends and family or when this is just not enough.

Yes, life will never be the same again, but the upheaval in the relationship is transient. With support and understanding for each other and from outside, it must be possible to build and strengthen love in the growing family. And no one, especially fathers, should underestimate the emotional involvement of men in pregnancy. It's real, but often kept under wraps.

Despite these warnings of dramatic change, there's an overwhelmingly good side to it. Be prepared, if you can, for joy! Many parents tell us that nothing compares with the joy of holding your child and the love that develops and grows between you as they grow.

Depression

We know from research that the health and development of new babies is affected adversely by depression in mothers. So far research has concentrated on detecting depression during pregnancy and giving treatment, but it must make sense to try to **prevent** depression in pregnancy. Depression is a very common and easily treated illness. We think that it would be logical to detect and treat depression as part of preparation for pregnancy. If you think you may be suffering from depression, consult your family doctor **before** becoming pregnant. There are several ways of treating depression. Counselling may help, or simply the support of friends or family. Cognitive therapy involves analysing thought patterns, finding ways of changing negative thoughts and understanding how these thoughts are linked to low moods. Being aware of these mental processes may allow sufferers to combat depression. Finally, antidepressant drugs are effective in treatment. A combination of all the above treatments may be needed.

If you're unsure about whether or not you are suffering from depression, try the questionnaire below:

Mark the answer that comes closest to how you have felt in the **last week**:

1. I have been able to laugh and see the funny side of things
    a) As much as I always could
    b) Not quite so much now
    c) Definitely not so much now
    d) Not at all

2. I have looked forward with enjoyment to things
    (a) As much as I ever did
    (b) Rather less than I used to
    (c) Definitely less than I used to
    (d) Hardly at all

3. I have blamed myself unnecessarily when things go wrong
    (a) Yes, most of the time
    (b) Yes, some of the time
    (c) Not very often
    (d) No, never

4. I have been anxious and worried for no good reason
    (a) No, not at all
    (b) Hardly ever
    (c) Yes, sometimes
    (d) Yes, very often

5. I have felt scared or panicky for no very good reason
    (a) Yes, quite a lot
    (b) Yes, sometimes
    (c) No, not much
    (d) No, not at all

6. Things have been getting on top of me
    (a) Yes, most of the time I haven't been able to cope at all
    (b) Yes, sometimes I haven't been coping as well as usual
    (c) No, most of the time I have coped quite well
    (d) No, I have been coping as well as ever

7. I have been so unhappy that I have had difficulty sleeping
    (a) Yes, most of the time
    (b) Yes, sometimes
    (c) Not very often
    (d) No, not at all

8. I have felt sad or miserable
    (a) Yes, most of the time
    (b) Yes, quite often
    (c) Not very often
    (d) No, not at all

9. I have been so unhappy that I have been crying
    (a) Yes, most of the time
    (b) Yes, quite often
    (c) Only occasionally
    (d) No, never

10. The thought of harming myself has occurred to me
    (a) Yes, quite often
    (b) Sometimes
    (c) Hardly ever
    (d) Never

SCORES
Questions 1, 2, 4: a–0, b–1, c–2, d–3
Questions 3, 5, 6, 7, 8, 9, 10: a–3, b–2, c–1, d–0
If you scored 12 or more, then you may be suffering from depression.

Anxiety

We are all familiar with the symptoms of anxiety – racing heart, sweating, rumbling tummy, shaking and many others. These symptoms are a normal response to situations in life with which we are unfamiliar. Pregnancy, or preparing for pregnancy, can be one such unfamiliar situation. First-time mothers may be expected to feel anxious about getting pregnant, about the pregnancy itself and the birth, and about caring for the new baby. Awareness of these fears can help in learning how to master them. Sometimes, however, these normal feelings get out of control, leading to loss of sleep and deterioration in health. If you feel that this is so for you, seek help, either from your doctor or from a local relaxation class or group.

PROBLEMS WITH GETTING PREGNANT

Having made the decision to have a baby, it can become frustrating and distressing when nothing happens.

How long should we wait?

Many factors are involved in conception and these vary for different people and at different times in their lives. As a guide, if there has been unprotected intercourse for a year, and no pregnancy has resulted, then it would be advisable to seek help from a family doctor. Of course for older women (approaching 40), there might be more pressure on time and perhaps six months would be reasonable.

Causes of Failure to Conceive

In order to start a pregnancy the following stages are needed:

- there must be normal sexual intercourse;
- the man must have sperm in sufficient numbers and of adequate quality;
- the woman must release an egg;
- the egg must be able to travel down the fallopian tube into the uterus;
- fertilisation of the egg by the sperm must occur during the journey from the ovary to the uterus;
- the fertilised egg must implant in the uterus.

Interference or problems at any of these stages may be the cause of failure to conceive.

Investigating Infertility

Most of the examinations and tests for problems with conception can be done by the family doctor (GP). Probably the majority of cases can be treated in General Practice; only a few needing expert intervention require treatment by specialists, and an even smaller number require the high-profile, expensive and sometimes controversial treatments such as IVF (In-vitro fertilisation).

The first step, as in all medical problems, is to 'take the history'. The doctor will ask for details about both partners, their past medical history and family history (both of which may already be known to a GP), their diet and lifestyle, how long they have been trying to conceive, and about the woman's menstrual cycle. The story gives a doctor a pretty good idea of what the problem might be. Examinations and special investigations confirm suspicions.

Next it must be established whether the man's sperm is adequate and whether the woman is ovulating.

Semen (sperm) analysis can be done by a doctor with a microscope but most use the local hospital laboratory. A sample produced by masturbation is examined under the microscope. The number of sperm are counted in a given area and their quality assessed. Sperm need to be 'mobile'. They literally swim through the uterus and into the fallopian tube to meet the egg. 'Poor quality sperm' lack this swimming ability.

There are several ways of determining whether ovulation is occurring, but the most reliable is to do hormone analysis. A rise in luteinising hormone in the middle of the cycle, and a rise in progesterone at the end, indicates ovulation. Other methods, such as temperature charts and examining cervical mucus, are unreliable and less used now. Ovulation predictor kits give reliable results. These can be used at home but they are expensive.

If there are adequate sperm and ovulation is occurring, then the problem must be a block between the cervix and the fallopian tube causing failure of sperm and egg to meet. This could be due to chronic infection at the cervix which the doctor would detect by examination and by sending samples to the bacteriology lab. Treatment could then be given. More likely, though, is a block in one or both fallopian tubes. To find this, special tests are needed. There are two possible ways. The first is laparoscopy with dye infusion, which involves a surgeon looking into the woman's abdomen with a laparoscope, a fibre optic instrument inserted through a small hole usually just below the umbilicus. At the same time dye is forced through the cervix and the operator can then see whether it spills out into the abdominal cavity, in which case the tube is open. The other way uses X-rays, and is called a salpingogram.

The advantages of laparoscopy, which is now the most commonly used method, are that the operator can see the dye directly and also look at the other organs for disease. The disadvantage is that a general anaesthetic is needed. The salpingogram is an indirect method, although it enables the radiologist to see the dye travelling inside the fallopian tubes. No anaesthetic is needed, but women complain that the procedure is uncomfortable and it exposes them to X-rays.

TREATING INFERTILITY

Quite often simple measures are all that is needed. Infertility clinics report that a large number of their patients conceive before any treatment has been given.

Male Problems

Smoking and alcohol in large amounts and heavy exercise all reduce sperm counts and sperm mobility. A good diet and healthy lifestyle can improve fertility for men. Work may be relevant especially if it involves exposure to chemicals – lead in particular.

Until quite recently research has concentrated on female infertility. So far, if there is complete azoospermia (absence of sperm altogether), there is no treatment available except artificial insemination with donor sperm (AID).

Female Problems

The same common sense about diet and lifestyle apply to ovulation. If ovulation is occurring then timing intercourse to coincide with release of the egg may help. In the past, women were given temperature charts to predict ovulation. This meant taking the temperature every day in the morning. When the temperature went up, that was the right time. More recently, ovulation kits using urine testing for hormones can predict ovulation.

> ## OVULATION
>
> **Evidence** Research shows that neither method of predicting ovulation is effective in producing pregnancies.
>
> **Opinion** We advise women to use a predictor kit to get an idea of when ovulation occurs in their cycle, but we feel that relying on predicting ovulation by either method involves far too much anxiety. We know that anxiety itself inhibits ovulation.

We think that the clinics' observation that many patients become pregnant before anything has been done has something to do with psychology. Anxiety causes increased levels of a hormone called prolactin, which plays a part in milk production after a birth. Prolactin inhibits ovulation. These facts may be useful to a couple who are having problems. Is there some way you can increase your relaxation, by doing exercises (there is a simple method in the next chapter), self-hypnosis, or yoga? Relaxation may tip the scales and result in a pregnancy before the doctor needs to be consulted.

If a woman is not ovulating then it is possible to stimulate ovulation by means of hormones. These include clomiphene which can be taken by mouth for five days before the middle of the cycle. Other hormones used in special hospital centres are given by injection or sniffed as a nasal spray. These are the ones that are associated with multiple births. Fallopian tube blockage usually needs surgery to repair. Often this is a major operation.

IVF, Gift etc

When none of the above treatments work, or when there is tube blockage which can't be repaired, the next step is some form of artificial fertilisation that is done in a special centre. There is no doubt that the successful birth of a baby following 'test tube' fertilisation (IVF) was a wonderful advance in science and the means of giving hope to many childless couples. There is a downside though. Even the best clinics using IVF, or GIFT (gamete intrafallopian transfer), publish their successful pregnancy rates as no higher than 40%. Women undergoing these treatments are subjected to enormous stresses, which the best clinics now recognise. They have introduced psychologists and counsellors to work alongside the specialists to help with this aspect of the treatment.

How it's done

IVF or GIFT or other methods all need to identify ovulation precisely so that the egg can be captured and fertilised. For IVF the fertilisation is done 'in vitro', which means outside the body. GIFT introduces sperm and egg together into the fallopian tube.

Ovulation can be allowed to occur naturally (the 'Natural Cycle Method') or it can be stimulated by injections of hormone, or nasal sprays of *buseralin*, or both. Either way, for about a week around the time of ovulation, the woman must travel each day to the clinic for either blood tests or ovum tracking by ultrasound scanning, or both. The scanning is usually done by the transvaginal route. When the egg is released it is captured by laparoscopy (under general anaesthetic) and fertilised with sperm, then replaced as a fertilised embryo in the case of IVF. Some clinics capture several eggs and fertilise them, keeping the resulting embryos frozen for future use. For many people this has moral and ethical implications.

Where to Go for Advice on Planning and Preparing for Pregnancy

Your General Practitioner (GP) should be able to give you all the information and check-ups you need to prepare for pregnancy. Some surgeries run special preconception clinics. If you don't have any luck at your own doctor's surgery, then your Local Health Authority will be able to tell you which doctors in your neighbourhood have a special interest in pregnancy or preconceptual care. Family Planning and Maternity services are treated as separate from General Medical Services, so in theory you could go to one doctor for advice about pregnancy and to another for your general medical care, but most people like to have a relationship of mutual trust with their doctors and feel that 'chopping and changing' might erode this. Equally, if doctors don't offer a particular service they can't complain if their patients go elsewhere to get it.

If you can't find a GP to give you the advice you need, your local Family Planning Clinic should provide the necessary expertise. Again, the Health Authority will advise on your nearest clinic.

Another source of advice is your Health Visitor who should be based either at the local GP's surgery or at the Community Health Clinic.

We believe that partnership between parents and professionals is the key to successful planning and preparation for pregnancy, and for pregnancy and birth itself. Part of preparation for pregnancy should be to begin to develop that partnership with a health professional, doctor, or midwife, whom you can get to know and trust.

Preparation for Pregnancy Checklist for Both Partners

- Doctor with Preconception Clinic or expertise?
- Advice on diet and exercise
- Smoking
- Alcohol
- Medicines and drugs
- Check Rubella immunisation
- Check for infections

CHAPTER TWO

EARLY PREGNANCY

....

THINGS TO DO

What to Eat – Nutrition in Pregnancy

Good nutrition is very important for both mother and baby. The same principles of a good diet while preparing for pregnancy apply to early pregnancy (see Chapter One). It is a matter of common sense that keeping up a good diet will help both mother and baby, and evidence from past 'natural experiments', such as the rationing during the Second World War which actually seemed to improve maternal and infant health, confirm this feeling. However, there is at present no research evidence to show definitely that any particular nutritional advice is beneficial to expectant mothers or their babies, **with one exception**. Folic acid supplements taken before pregnancy and during very early pregnancy help prevent spina bifida (see Chapter One). Folic acid is found in green vegetables and fruit so it makes sense to include plenty of these in a mother's diet.

Exercise

Gentle exercise is good for mother and baby, especially exercise in water – this can be swimming or exercises done in a pool. Many areas have aqua-natal classes and these are run by midwives, especially for expectant mothers, at local swimming pools. The midwives will have all the information about these classes.

EXERCISE IN WATER

Evidence Research has shown that such exercise is good for swollen legs (oedema) which occurs later in pregnancy, and also reduces blood pressure.

It's a good idea for mothers to start exercising early, but as with all exercise at any stage of life, it's sensible to start gently and build up the amount of exercise gradually. It's perfectly OK to continue with most kinds of regular exercise during pregnancy. The important principles to remember are:

– progesterone, a hormone which is increased in pregnancy, softens ligaments. There is a useful purpose for this in preparing the pelvis for labour, but it may mean that ligament strains occur more easily during pregnancy, so exercise which involves a lot of bending and stretching and twisting should be done with care.
– in later pregnancy as the weight is thrown forward, extra care of the back needs to be taken (see later).

Some Exercises for Early Pregnancy

You can do exercises in early pregnancy which do not involve strain on muscles or joints, but still burn up energy (aerobic exercise). These can even be done while sitting. We'll describe some simple exercises which are safe to do at home, but better still, go to an exercise class run by a qualified exercise teacher. Sometimes these take place at the local maternity hospital, especially for pregnant mothers. Ask your midwife.

It's not necessary to expend lots of energy (or money) on hard 'work-outs' in a gym with expensive equipment. Gentle exercise done at home can really improve health and well-being.

Getting in the right position (posture) is important. If you're sitting down, make sure your feet are flat on the ground, legs uncrossed and your back is straight and tummy pulled in. This is a good posture for sitting at any time. These exercises can be done standing or sitting, or even in the bath, where the buoyancy of the water adds to relaxation and improves muscle tone.

1.   Shoulders and neck rolling
Loosen your shoulders first before your neck.

Lift one arm above your head and stretch over your head, then bring it down, keeping the arm straight, but relaxed. Repeat this about eight times, and then do the same with the other arm.

Roll your head to one side, feeling a slight stretch on the opposite side, then roll it around to the other side. Repeat this on each side for about eight times.

2.   Biceps curls
Make a fist with one hand. Slowly pull your hand up towards your shoulder and then relax. Repeat about eight times and then repeat with the other arm.

3.   For the chest and shoulders
Make a fist again with both hands and then bring them slowly round to meet behind your back. Breathe in as you do this. Then relax. Repeat eight times. This is best done standing but can also be done on a low-backed chair.

4.   The pelvic tilt
This is a good exercise for strengthening the abdominal muscles. Lie on the floor with legs bent and feet flat on the floor. Pulling in your tummy, tilt your pelvis up towards you so that you see it dip in the middle and feel your lower back pushing into the floor. Relax and repeat four times. This can also be done standing up. In later pregnancy when the tummy is larger and heavier it is best to get support by leaning backwards against a wall. If standing, keep your knees soft and relaxed and the same distance apart as your hips.

5.   For the legs
Sit on a chair with one leg bent. Bring the other leg up to knee height with toes pulled towards your face. Hold for a moment, then relax. Repeat this eight times, then do the same with the other leg. Remember to keep your knees relaxed.

6.   Heel and toe pointing for the ankles
This is useful to keep the ankles supple and especially if you have swelling

which can be uncomfortable. Sitting on a chair, with the left foot flat, put your right heel to the floor and then your right toes. Repeat this eight times and then repeat with the other foot. Placing a hand under your calf to support it, make circles with your foot – eight times in one direction and then reverse, then repeat with the other foot.

Sex

Being pregnant makes a difference to both partners but every couple reacts differently. Some find that pregnancy makes no difference while others seem to lose sexual desire during pregnancy. The reasons for this are a complicated mixture of physical and emotional factors. Changes in hormone levels and body size and shape may affect the mother while fear of some ill effect on the baby may affect the father. Sex is actually perfectly safe throughout pregnancy unless there is a particular risk of bleeding or miscarriage. Some experimentation with position may be necessary as the baby gets bigger. Many find the 'spoons' position, with the woman lying on her side and the partner tucked closely behind, is the most comfortable. Can you be gentle and considerate to each other and if intercourse is not possible, enjoy a cuddle?

Work

There is no need for employers to know straight away about the pregnancy, but if you are working in a situation that may be hazardous to the baby, then it's best to tell your employer as soon as possible in order to reduce the risk.

Jobs that may expose mothers to risk are:

Health Service Workers

- Radiographers and people working in radiotherapy departments may be exposed to ionising radiation. There are strict controls over the exposure of pregnant women to such radiation under the UK Ionising Radiation Regulations (1985).
- Nurses and other staff working in oncology units should take extra precautions over the handling of cytotoxic drugs.

◆ People working in operating theatres where they may be exposed to anaesthetic gases should also be given special consideration, though no regulations govern this and there is doubt about the evidence of any hazard.

Workers in the chemical industry or who may use chemicals at work

◆ Lead is highly toxic to babies and is strictly controlled by the Lead Regulations which prohibit pregnant women from working with it. Large numbers of women work in assembly processes involving lead, such as in battery manufacture or enamelling.
◆ Mercury – organic mercury is toxic to babies, but rarely used in the UK. It may be present in seed dressings. Dental nurses mix mercury amalgams and should take care, but there is no evidence at present that this is hazardous.
◆ Ethylene oxide is used as a sterilising agent in hospitals. There is some evidence that it causes spontaneous miscarriage in workers using it.
◆ Organic solvents may be associated with fetal abnormalities and they are also excreted in breast milk and may be hazardous to breast-fed babies. Examples of these are xylene, toluene, styrene, alcohols of different kinds, and ketones.

If in doubt about any kind of chemical which you may be exposed to at work, you should ask the Safety Officer to look up the Data Sheet on that chemical to check on its safety.

Visual Display Units (VDUs)

There is controversy about the safety of working with VDUs when pregnant. The worry is that the low levels of radiation emitted by such machines may increase the risk of miscarriage. The evidence at present does not confirm such a risk, but because of the element of doubt which still remains, many employers will find alternative jobs for pregnant workers (see also Chapter One).

Heavy manual work

This is associated with a higher risk of miscarriage and premature labour. If you are concerned about your job in this respect, seek the support of your midwife and doctor in asking for a reduction in your hours of work or a transfer to lighter duties. When thinking about the physical strain of a job, women should also take into consideration the work they may do in housework and childcare, both of which may also expose them to toxic chemicals (eg, pesticides and household spray cleaners).

If you're working in a safe job which you enjoy, then you may want to plan to carry on work up to 29 weeks or beyond that. At 26 weeks, mothers are entitled to a 'certificate of expected confinement' also known as a MAT B1 which confirms the expected date of the birth and must be signed by a midwife or doctor. This document must be sent or given to your employer three weeks before you intend to stop work in order to claim Statutory Maternity Pay (SMP). It's a good idea to look at your contract of employment if you have one, or find out from your employer about maternity leave. There is a legal right for women to have maternity leave and to return to their job afterwards, but there are conditions which apply to this, and it is best to check these out early on so you can make plans about when it would be best to stop work. Employers may have their own maternity leave schemes but the minimum required of them by law is that women who have been employed for more than six months are entitled to 18 weeks paid maternity leave. Of this, 12 weeks will be on full pay and six weeks on half pay. After that the job must be held open for one year. Trade unions should be able to advise on mothers' maternity leave and employment rights.

If you have not been working enough to get SMP then you can claim a basic Maternity Allowance, using form MAT B1.

Factors influencing your decision on when to stop work may be:

– your state of health;
– any complications of pregnancy such as pre-eclampsia (complicated high blood pressure);
– the nature of the work – heavy jobs become more difficult as the pregnancy progresses;
– will you want to return to work afterwards?

Maternity Leave Checklist

◆ When should I stop work?
◆ Collect MAT B1 at 26 weeks.

- How shall I arrange the 18 weeks paid leave?
- When do I plan to return to work?
- Does my employer have their own scheme which is more advantageous? Get details.

Other Entitlements

- **Free Dental Care** Take advantage of this. While you are pregnant, and for one year after the birth, you can have all your NHS dental care free.
- **Free Prescriptions** You don't pay prescription charges while pregnant and for a year after the birth. A form is needed which your family doctor, or midwife can issue. You must fill it in and send it to your Local Health Authority who will issue a certificate exempting you from prescription charges.

Going to 'the Doctor's'

For most women, the most natural first contact with the health services in pregnancy is their family doctor. The GP may be able to confirm pregnancy and encourages women to attend as soon as they know that they are pregnant.

How Do You Know You're Pregnant?

The most obvious sign is a missed period, but this is not completely reliable because sometimes periods can be missed for other reasons, and not everyone's cycle is the regular 28 days. Bleeding can occur in early pregnancy which may seem like a period and can cause more confusion. Other signs are breast tenderness, and a tendency to want to go to the toilet to pass urine more frequently. Nausea (feeling sick) and feeling faint may also be early signs. To confirm suspicions, a pregnancy test is the best step. This can be done at the GP's surgery at no charge, using either NHS laboratories or testing kits in the surgery, or for a fee by your local pharmacist. Home-testing kits can be bought from the chemist. These kits are now very reliable. All tests use the same principle – the detection of a hormone in urine. The hormone is produced when the baby embeds itself in the wall of the womb, from the part which later becomes the placenta.

Working Out When the Baby is Due

Midwives and doctors like to work out an Expected Date of Delivery (EDD) from the date of the mother's last period. You can do this yourself if you're sure of the date. Take the first day of your last period and add on seven days and nine months. For example, if your period started on 12th May, the EDD would be 19th February next year. *But* the EDD can be very misleading. It is normal for the baby to be born at any time between 38 and 42 weeks after the last period.

We prefer to give mothers a range of dates when the baby is due. It helps planning better. It seems to us that too much emphasis is placed on the EDD by both professionals and mothers. Again, between 38 and 42 weeks is normal. That means there's a whole month during which the baby may be born. We also know that 70% of mothers actually give birth after the EDD, but everyone's anxiety levels seem to rise after the EDD has passed. To be realistic about planning your life and to avoid getting anxious, work out your EDD, then add two weeks either side. Get this range of dates fixed in your mind. For example, if your period was 12th May, making the EDD 19th February, your baby is due between 5th February and 5th March. Even then there is still some flexibility about the date.

TIP

Normal pregnancy lasts from 38 to 42 weeks. So don't fix on one date, have a month in mind.

SO YOU'RE PREGNANT – WHAT NOW?

Things to Avoid

The baby's development is complete by 12 weeks. All that happens after 12 weeks is that the baby grows. So the first three months is really a crucial time. Many factors in the baby's immediate environment (in the womb) can influence its development. There are some we know and probably many more we don't know. The ones we know about are infection, drugs (medicinal and non-medicinal) and, of course, alcohol and tobacco. The perfect solution is to avoid all these things in the first three months of pregnancy, but perfection is rarely possible, so common sense is needed.

SMOKING

Smoking stops nutrition from reaching the growing baby (see also Chapter One).

Evidence We know from research that babies born to mothers who smoke are smaller on average than those born to non-smokers. The brain as well as the rest of the body tends to be smaller and we know that not only does this increase the risk to the newborn baby, but also that later on reading ability is reduced in the children born to mothers who smoke in pregnancy. Passive smoking has a similar effect.

The common sense plan then must be not to smoke at all in pregnancy and to avoid smoky places, and to get your partner to stop as well even if only for a short while.

Alcohol

We know that alcohol affects the growth and development of babies (see Chapter One) and the best advice must be: don't drink at all in pregnancy; if you must drink, then at least give your baby a chance during that first vital three months.

ALCOHOL

Evidence Drinking occasionally in pregnancy does not harm the baby. This means less than ten units a week, provided the whole lot is not consumed in one go. One unit of alcohol is half a pint of normal strength beer, cider, or lager, a quarter of a pint of strong beer or lager, one glass of wine, one small glass of sherry or a single measure of spirit. Very heavy drinking can result in the baby getting a condition known as *fetal alcohol syndrome*. Babies with this condition have problems with their sight and hearing and will have learning difficulties. They are more likely to be small at birth and to fail to grow properly. The risks of the baby getting this syndrome are increased if the mother is also a smoker and has a poor diet.

Opinion If possible, women should not drink at all in pregnancy.

Mothers who are worried about their drinking, or feel that they should cut down but find it difficult, should get help. The midwife or GP will be glad to help and advise about drinking. Help can also be found from other agencies:

National Alcohol Helpline: 0345 320202 (local rates)

Alcohol Concern
Waterbridge House
32–36 Loman Street
London SE1 OEE
(0171 928 7377)

Alcoholics Anonymous
General Service Office
Stonebow House
Stonebow
York Y01 2NJ
(01904 644026)

DAWN
(Drugs and Alcohol Women's Network)
C/O GLAAS
30–31 Great Sutton Street
London ECIV ODX
(0171 253 6221)

Infection

Viruses

Some well-known viruses can affect the baby's development, especially *German measles* (rubella), *measles, mumps* and *chicken pox*. Less well known but equally common are the *Coxsackie* viruses and *herpes*. *Cytomegalovirus* (CMV) can also cause serious illness in a baby and can affect development. CMV causes an illness like glandular fever. It can be chronically present in people on immunosuppressive drugs or whose immunity is severely impaired due to chronic illness.

Most people have now been immunised against rubella (but every woman planning a pregnancy should have her immunity to rubella checked before conception – see Chapter One). Many women will also have been immunised against measles and mumps, which are disappearing from our population. Most of us had chicken pox as children. The best advice though is, if you know someone who has one of these virus infections, stay away, especially during the first three months of pregnancy.

Infection of the Urinary Tract

This is the most common complication of pregnancy. Three to eight per cent of women are recorded to have infection. However, it is often unrecognised because it may not cause symptoms or the symptoms (running frequently to the toilet, for example) get confused with the normal symptoms of pregnancy. The risk with infection of the bladder is that it may spread to infect the kidney causing pyelonephritis, which has potential long term effects on the health of the mother, and potential effects on the baby. Pyelonephritis affects about one in a hundred pregnancies. It can be treated with antibiotics. The symptoms are backache and a fever, sometimes with the urine stinging or burning. If you get any of these, or you are unsure, consult your doctor or midwife as soon as possible.

Listeria

This is a bacterium which can cause miscarriage, stillbirth or premature labour. It is found widely in the environment, especially in the soil and on plants, and it is notoriously found in unpasteurised cheese (especially soft cheese such as Brie and Camembert). These should be avoided, especially in the first three months of pregnancy. Supermarkets are now very fussy about food hygiene but there have been instances of listeria found in pre-packed salads, especially if they cannot be washed before eating. A council of perfection for the pregnant mother is to eat only hard cheese, such as Cheshire and Cheddar, or cottage cheese, and to eat only salads and vegetables that have been prepared at home and washed thoroughly.

Toxoplasma

This is a parasite which infects animals and humans. It can result in congenital infection of the baby with serious results – effects on the eyes and brain. The risk of severe disease in the baby is higher if infection is acquired early in pregnancy. The most common form of infection for the baby, however, is Subclinical Congenital Toxoplasmosis where the mother is infected in later pregnancy. The baby is apparently normal at birth but weeks, months or even years later, develops eye problems or hydrocephalus, a condition of too much fluid surrounding the brain.

People can only be infected once, so if you are immune there is no risk. Infection is usually mild, with symptoms of a slight fever and joint pains like 'flu, and most people don't even know that they have had it. Raw meat and cat litter are the two most common sources of infection, so common sense will avoid trouble. Other sources of infection are the soil and unpasteurised milk. Don't eat raw or undercooked meat and wash your hands carefully after handling raw meat. Wear gloves for gardening and handling cat litter. Wash fruit and vegetables thoroughly and avoid unpasteurised milk and milk products. Children's sand pits or boxes should be covered if outside, to prevent soiling by cats.

Salmonella

This is a food poisoning bacterium which contaminates food such as poultry and eggs, and also cream and dairy products. It is destroyed by thorough cooking. Salmonella causes diarrhoea and vomiting which is unpleasant for anyone, but some infected people become carriers; although the body will eventually clear the infection naturally, there is no treatment that will eradicate the bacteria. Small babies are very prone to infection and may rapidly become dehydrated and ill because of salmonella, so we should all try to prevent mothers from carrying the germ. Avoid raw or undercooked eggs. Avoid raw eggs in food such as home-made mayonnaise, or mousse, or ice cream. Always cook poultry and meat well and if you reheat food, make sure that it is really piping hot and never reheat more than once. Cooked and chilled chicken from supermarkets should also be avoided in pregnancy.

Liver

This is mostly a healthy food to eat but if you're pregnant, it's best avoided. The reason for this is that it contains high levels of vitamin A which is a good thing for most of us most of the time, but for the baby there may be too much, resulting in damage to the brain and nervous system.

Antenatal Care

We are at the beginning of a revolution in antenatal care. Dr Ian Chalmers, formerly the director of the National Perinatal Epidemiology Unit, writes: 'It is uncertain which routinely performed procedures are effective in promoting the health of pregnant women or their babies. In many areas of care, the available experimentally derived data are inadequate to support strong inferences about their effects and in others there are no data available.' In other words, we don't know which measurements and tests are useful and which are not.

Antenatal care really started seriously in the 1920s, with the good idea that looking after the health of pregnant women before birth would help to reduce maternal deaths. Later the focus changed to reducing deaths of babies. Fewer babies die during or immediately after birth now and deaths of mothers are thankfully rare, but during the last 70 years, other changes in society have occurred which are probably much more important in improving health than antenatal care. We are all wealthier, eat better and have better housing.

We believe that education and support for mothers are more important in antenatal care than clinical measurement, and that tests and examinations should be done only when there is a reason to do them – ie not just for routine or because of habitual procedures. For now, what most mothers can expect at a hospital or GP's surgery is to see a midwife or a doctor for a brief chat about how they are feeling, have their blood pressure checked, their urine tested, and in some clinics to be weighed.

A lot of heat is generated by obstetricians about these procedures, some believing, for example, that blood pressure measurement is important and that this should be done every week, while others believe that fewer measurements are necessary. Almost everyone is now agreed, from the evidence, that weighing women has no value at all, yet we were at a conference recently when a highly respected professor of obstetrics gave a lecture, including all the evidence that weighing was a waste of time, but then stated that he still insisted on weighing women attending his own clinic!

At an antenatal clinic blood tests for anaemia and blood groups will be taken at various stages of pregnancy. Screening for spina bifida and Downs' syndrome by blood tests and ultrasound scanning will be offered. We'll discuss screening in detail later. A midwife or doctor will probably then examine the abdomen to check that the baby is growing, that its heart is beating normally and, later in pregnancy, that it is in the right position for birth. Although most clinics have not moved away from a 'medical model' of care, there is a general move towards a less clinical approach and giving more attention to the needs of mothers. The more women ask for this, and ask questions of the professionals, the faster change will come about.

Most antenatal care can now be carried out in the community, reducing the need for women to attend hospital. This was a recommendation of the 'Changing Childbirth' report in 1994. Even if some hospital care is needed, most antenatal visits can be made to the GP's surgery and midwives will arrange home visits to mothers for some check-ups, especially the first or 'booking' visit. Very few of our mothers attend the hospital. In the future, we think that only women with difficult medical problems will need to go to hospital for antenatal care.

It is a good idea to think through where you would like most of your care to take place before going to the doctor's to make the arrangements.

Checklist for Antenatal Care

- ◆ Any serious medical problems which may need hospital care?
- ◆ Where to have most care? Home, GP's surgery or hospital?
- ◆ GP willing or able to provide care?
- ◆ Community midwife willing or able to provide care?

Early Problems in Pregnancy

The first three months are the worst! This is often true, but not always; some mothers have no problems at all, others experience sickness and other symptoms throughout pregnancy.

Morning Sickness

This may not happen only in the morning. No one knows what causes women to feel sick or to be sick in early pregnancy but it is quite common in the first three months. For most women it gets better after 12–14 weeks. Some doctors will prescribe antihistamine tablets (travel sickness pills) to relieve the sickness but there is no firm evidence that these are totally safe for the baby and there may be side effects for the mother such as drowsiness and blurred vision.

Acupressure at the wrist has been proved to be effective in research studies. This is a relatively easy technique to learn and your doctor or midwife may be able to use it. If not, local acupuncturists or reflexologists will be listed in Yellow Pages (or contact the British Acupuncture Association and Register). If it's not possible to find a professional to demonstrate acupressure, try finding the 'P6' Neguin point for yourself and either apply gentle sustained pressure with your thumb for two minutes, or do small circulatory massage movements with your thumb or first finger on this point for two minutes. The P6 point is found on the wrist, just above the crease, in the middle, between the two prominent tendons in the wrist.

Homoeopathic remedies may also be helpful and are perfectly safe for both mother and baby. Nux vomica and Ipecac are probably the two most commonly used remedies for 'morning sickness'. Pulsatilla and Sepia may also be tried (see checklist). Low potency tablets of one of these could be tried and are available from the local pharmacy, who may be able to advise on their use. Some doctors and midwives have experience in homoeopathy. Local lay homoeopaths can be found in Yellow Pages or by phoning the Society of Homoeopaths (address given at end of chapter). Reflexology may also help morning sickness (see Chapter Five).

Checklist for Morning Sickness Remedies

- Use *Nux vomica* if nausea and retching is relieved by being sick; you suffer from sour belching and retching, or from indigestion and heartburn; you feel a 'knot' in the stomach; you feel irritable.
- Use *Ipecac* if nausea and retching is not relieved by being sick.
- Use *Pulsatilla* if nausea is worse after eating or drinking; it feels better in fresh air and in company; you feel weepy and moody and need comforting.
- Use *Sepia* if nausea comes and goes and is worse in the mornings and for the smell and thought of food; you have an empty sinking feeling in the stomach which is temporarily relieved by eating; you feel as if everything is too much trouble, but surprisingly better for exercise.

Tiredness
Unfortunately tiredness is normal in early pregnancy. There has been no research on this problem. Tiredness does not usually mean that the sufferer is anaemic. Common sense measures help. Rest is the sensible thing to do when tired; perhaps this symptom has a useful purpose and enforces rest when it is needed. If you feel tired, pamper yourself and try to get your partner to do the same. It will give him a sense of usefulness if he knows that he has to look after you a little more than usual in pregnancy.

Heartburn
This affects two out of three pregnant women and can be very uncomfortable and distressing, especially as it often gets worse when you lie

down, and so disturbs sleep. It can start in early pregnancy, but becomes more of a problem as the baby gets bigger. Avoid fatty or spicy foods, and try taking antacids such as milk of magnesia or ask the doctor for a prescription. Strangely, dilute acids such as citric acid (lemon juice or other fruit juices) often bring relief while milk makes it worse. Homoeopathic Causticum may help. Some exercises may help to relieve or prevent heartburn – see Chapter Five.

Constipation
This is more of a problem in late pregnancy, but to avoid it, start following a good wholefood diet from the beginning with plenty of fibre, fruit, vegetables and wholemeal bread. Increase your fluid intake, especially water. Avoid taking iron tablets unless you are really anaemic.

Homoeopathic remedies that may help are:

– *Bryonia* if you also have a headache which is worse for the slightest movement.
– *Nux vomica* if you 'can't go' although you frequently get the urge.
– *Sepia* if your stomach feels full and there is a feeling of a lump in the rectum even after going to the toilet.
– *Sulphur* if you have piles that itch and burn, and/or if you generally feel worse for heat.

Urinary Frequency and Infection
One of the first signs of pregnancy may be having to go to the toilet more often to pass urine. It is not certain why this happens in early pregnancy. It can also be a problem towards the end of pregnancy when the baby's head presses on the bladder. In the first three months there is no real remedy but the situation improves as the baby grows. Avoiding bladder stimulants like tea, coffee and Coke (and also alcohol) may help. Frequent passing of urine may be a symptom of urinary tract infection which is one of the most common complications of pregnancy, affecting about one in a hundred pregnancies. Other symptoms of UTI are a burning sensation when passing urine and discomfort in the lower part of the tummy where the bladder is. Backache may also be a symptom of UTI. Up to eight women in a hundred harbour bacteria in the bladder during pregnancy without knowing it. (Technically asymptomatic bacteriuria.)

URINARY TRACT INFECTION

Evidence Studies have shown that treatment prevents complications and leads to a better outcome for mother and baby, so routine urine testing is carried out in antenatal clinics.

Psychological Problems

Stress – the nature of it

Stress itself is not a disease. We all need a little stress. Without it we would fail to perform even simple tasks. It is part of our natural defence against danger and helps us when we need to produce some extra effort for something. For example, if we have to run to catch a bus, our adrenaline goes up when we see the bus arriving (literally – levels of this hormone increase in the bloodstream). This adrenaline causes several effects. Our heart rate increases, we breathe faster and fat is freed in our blood stream as a fuel to aid the extra work we will need to do in running. These sort of changes also happen when we are under stress which requires less physical effort, such as preparing for an interview for a job, or for an exam, or approaching the hospital for a check-up.

Other effects of stress which are less helpful in a 'running for the bus' situation are increased activity in the bowels, which can cause diarrhoea, and also increased tone in the bladder which produces the feeling of wanting to pass urine. Many of us in the twentieth century, both men and women, seem to be living in a constant 'running for a bus' situation. This is when stress becomes bad for us. Remember, we need a little bit, it's useful and helps us in emergencies, but too much stress, in fact, reduces the ability to perform – as any musician will tell you.

Causes of stress

Change

Many of our 1990s' stress problems relate to the rapid pace of change taking place all around us. A lot of us have been removed from our roots – our home towns and families, and from traditional sources of support – friends and family. There is overcrowding in our towns and on our roads and there is uncertainty about job security and about relationships which is manifested in a high divorce rate. Some researchers have produced a scale for stressful events with the death of a husband or wife rated as the most stressful at 100 points, divorce at 73, dismissal from work at 47 and Christmas at 12 points. Pregnancy rates at 40 points on this scale, and the birth of a child at 39. A score of over 300 in a twelve-month period indicates a major crisis. Very often we don't realise how much we are subject to stressful events, and rating scales such as this can help to focus attention. For example, a woman becoming pregnant for the first time may have a number of other stressful events or changes to cope with during the same year:

Marriage	50
Pregnancy	40
Change in income	38
Moving home	20
Trouble with in-laws	28
Stopping work	47
Change in sleep	17
Change in eating	15
Christmas	12
TOTAL	267

We do not always have control over the events going on around us, but we may be able to change the way we react to such stresses in order to minimise the effects. It can be worthwhile stopping to ask whether there are options or choices we can make that can alter what is happening, but which we are ignoring. This applies especially to pregnancy because so often the choice is taken from mothers by professionals making decisions 'for the best interests of the baby'.

Lifestyle

This, on the other hand, is something over which we have much more control. Our habits and behaviour influence our response to stress. Smoking and alcohol, as well as being bad for the baby during pregnancy, are also contributors to stress. This is unfortunate because we often turn to these as props when we are under stress. 'Have a cigarette to calm you down', or 'That's terrible, let me get you a drink', are common reactions from well-meaning friends to stressful situations. Such responses will only make things worse.

Support from our friends and family, those closest to us, is what is really needed in stressful situations. Mothers in pregnancy need this more than most people, yet they may not get what they need because everyone expects them to be happy and healthy. The imminent arrival of the baby is seen as a 'happy event', which of course it is, but it is also an enormous change in the lives of a couple. So we want to encourage mothers to talk about their hopes and fears, their worries and problems. Talk to someone who is close and will understand. Husbands or partners are the closest and most accessible sources of support, but they may not notice the stress. Often mothers tell us that they are being horrid to their partners and attribute it to changes in their hormones. This is not likely to be the case. Most partners will be understanding and supportive if only they are asked. Our advice is, if you are feeling stressed and in need of support, choose a time to ask carefully – when you both have time to sit and talk. Ask for what you want directly – 'I am feeling worried about ―― and I need some help. Will you help me, please?' – rather than indirect questions or statements which may be misinterpreted. If this still doesn't work, then seek help elsewhere, from family or friends or from your professional advisers – midwife or GP or Health Visitor – but don't bottle it all up.

Inside Ourselves

We've discussed stress and ways of dealing with it in terms of external factors, but probably the most important elements in the causes and treatment of stress are those inside ourselves – our feelings and emotions and the way we think about ourselves.

Depression

If you feel depressed or in low spirits, it is important to seek help sooner rather than later. If you're not sure whether the way you are feeling is depression, then go through the checklist in Chapter One.

Asserting Yourself

From the beginning of pregnancy, through all the months of antenatal care, and right up to the birth, a mother can be vulnerable. Changes are happening to your body which you may find difficult to understand, professionals will be giving advice and recommending things for you to do; for example having tests, altering your lifestyle, or choosing a certain type of care. In labour, a mother can be especially vulnerable. **It's your body and it's your baby**, so it should be you that makes the decisions. You need information to do this. We hope you can find much of what you need in this book, but a better source is asking the midwife or doctor who is looking after you. In this possibly bewildering situation how can you:

a) ask the questions and get the information you need to make choices?
b) stand up for yourself and your baby in the decisions you have made?

We encourage our mothers to be **assertive**. This means being *independent*, having a mind of your own and making your own decisions. It also means being *decisive*, being definite about what you expect from other people, from those professionals giving you care in pregnancy and at the birth, and from your husband or partner and family. Be definite about your own priorities for your antenatal care and what you would like to happen at the birth. If you are not naturally this sort of a person, then it would be a good opportunity to develop assertiveness skills during the pregnancy, as these can be learnt. They will be helpful to you during antenatal care, when you are in labour and for life afterwards. An assertive person is not aggressive. Aggression usually produces a defensive reaction – it is more effective to decide what your priorities and needs are, and to state them quietly and calmly but firmly and repeatedly if necessary. You can practise doing this with friends or in a group.

Imagine this everyday situation:

You are tired. When you get home, everything is in a mess. Your husband is reading the newspaper. How do you get help clearing up? Do you:

a) run in, grab the newspaper and shout 'who the hell do you think you are?'
b) do the clearing up yourself, all the time thinking how inconsiderate he is, then go and cook tea.
c) mutter 'Look at this mess, I don't know how you can be so inconsiderate,' then clear up yourself and cook the tea, making sure that everyone feels guilty.

None of these responses give a specific statement of what you actually want. The most effective way to get help is usually to ask for it directly:

'I'm tired and I'd like you to help me get tea ready. I'd like you to do the washing up.'

The three skills which are effective and assertive are:

1. Decide what you want or feel, and say it specifically and directly (straight out).
2. Stick to your statement, repeating it, if necessary, again and again.
3. Deal with responses without being side-tracked.

This can often mean showing that you have heard the other person's point of view while still maintaining your own. 'I know you want to read the paper, but I'd still like you to help me with the tea.'

If you can imagine possible difficult situations that you might meet during your pregnancy or birth, then it might help you to deal with them by practising these simple tricks. A friend can help by playing the part of the other person.

Colleges of Education often run assertiveness training courses, so if you think you have a problem asserting yourself, try to attend one. Your family doctor may also be able to arrange help from a counsellor or psychologist.

Threatened Miscarriage

Miscarriage is sadly very common and affects up to one in three pregnancies. Before pregnancy testing became so accurate (in the last 15 years), many pregnancies probably miscarried without being recognised. Miscarriage certainly causes great distress to families. Although a small amount of bleeding from the vagina in early pregnancy is quite a common event and may not signify any serious problem, any bleeding at this stage should be considered a threatened miscarriage. The heavier the bleeding, the more likely the baby is to miscarry. Colicky pain in the tummy may accompany the bleeding. If bleeding occurs, however slight, the doctor should be consulted as soon as is practical. Very heavy bleeding with clots is an emergency which may even be life-threatening to the mother and immediate medical help should be summoned. If you go to the doctor's surgery because of bleeding in early pregnancy, you should expect the doctor to perform or arrange for an ultrasound scan. This is the best indicator of whether the baby is alive and well. If the scan shows that the baby is alive, then no further action need be taken. It makes sense to rest, and to avoid intercourse and really vigorous sports, but complete bed rest is certainly not necessary.

If the scan shows that the baby has died, then two courses of action are possible. If the bleeding stops completely then no further action may be necessary, except perhaps a repeat scan to make sure that there are no 'products of conception' left in the uterus. If the bleeding continues, then the obstetrician in charge of the case may recommend 'evacuation of products of conception' (EPOC). A brief general anaesthetic is given, the cervix is dilated and remaining tissue removed from the uterus. This usually results in the bleeding stopping. Advice is often given not to conceive for three months following a miscarriage but there is no evidence to support this advice.

MISCARRIAGE

Evidence There is no evidence that any form of treatment or precautions taken by the mother or her medical attendants will make any difference to the outcome or prevent a miscarriage.

Miscarriage can be a very emotionally traumatic experience for a woman and for her partner. Men are expected to shrug off such events and notoriously conceal their feelings. In addition to the trauma of the event itself, there is often a sense of loss for both partners and it is important for both to be understanding and supportive of each other. Women often say to us that they felt they knew their babies even at this early stage of pregnancy and that they grieve almost as though they had lost a grown child. Unfortunately, people often seem to be insensitive to the loss involved in a miscarriage. The advice 'better luck next time' is not really very helpful. Potential mothers and fathers should allow themselves, and be allowed by others, to grieve for the loss of a child after a miscarriage. Fathers may feel a great sense of deflation after initial excitement about the prospect of a baby. A miscarriage is a stressful event which can strain a couple's relationship. A determination to support each other and emerge stronger from the experience may be helpful.

Some positive encouragement may be drawn though, from a purely mathematical point of view. If miscarriage affects one in three pregnancies, then the chance of miscarrying once is one in three, the chance of two in a row is one in nine and the chance of three in a row is one in 27. This assumes that no biological factor is affecting the ability to sustain a pregnancy.

Not much is known about the factors which affect miscarriage but research is now growing for those women who suffer repeated miscarriages. Progress has been slow since the discovery, in the early eighties, that for a small number of women, incompatibility of tissue type between male and female partners is a treatable problem. Some specialists concentrate on research into this area and if you suffer from repeated miscarriages it may be a good idea to ask your doctor for referral to such a centre. Another very rare but treatable problem is the antiphospholipid syndrome which not only causes repeated miscarriage but also affects blood clotting and causes respiratory problems for sufferers. Repeated miscarriage in this condition responds to treatment with low-dose aspirin.

When miscarried fetuses can be found and examined, a proportion of them (about 30%) have chromosome abnormalities. A small number of people carry chromosome abnormalities without being aware of it, so chromosome analysis may be offered to couples (both male and female partners) who have experienced repeated miscarriage.

However, many women feel that with the chances of a cure still remote, they prefer to rely on nature.

Twins

About one in a hundred pregnancies is a twin pregnancy. The incidence of triplets and higher numbers has increased in recent years because of the use of hormones to stimulate ovulation. The chance of twins for mothers taking clomiphene (Clomid) to stimulate ovulation, is about seven per hundred pregnancies. For triplets it is about five per thousand, compared to one in ten thousand pregnancies where no fertility drug has been used.

Twins are now diagnosed early in pregnancy because of ultrasound scanning. They are often spotted on a scan before the mother shows signs of carrying twins, the most obvious sign being that she is 'too big for dates'. Sometimes mothers are told that they are carrying twins early on and then a later scan shows only one baby. It is assumed then that one baby has miscarried. This can happen without the mother being aware, but sometimes there may be bleeding with the miscarriage.

Twins can be identical or non-identical. About one in three twin births results in identical twins. Identical twins come from the same egg which has been fertilised by a sperm and then divided into two to produce two embryos. They are always of the same sex, half of those born being boy pairs and half girl pairs. Non-identical twins result from two eggs which are released either from the same ovary or one from each ovary and which are then fertilised by two different sperms. This fertilisation usually occurs at the same time, but there can be a gap of three or four days. There have been rare cases where twins were proven to have different fathers.

Non-identical twins run in families – but only in the mother's. A woman with non-identical twins on her mother's side of the family has a higher chance of twins. Identical twins do not run in families. The chance of twins increases with each pregnancy and as the woman gets older.

The signs of twins are:

– a uterus which is 'large for dates', in other words when the midwife or doctor feels the mother's abdomen, the uterus feels bigger than it should do for the length of the pregnancy.
– weight gain. Mothers themselves notice this first – they seem to be putting on too much weight.
– too many 'fetal parts' – there are lots of kicks and movements from twice as many arms and legs.

If you notice any of these signs, don't be afraid to question whether you might be expecting twins. An ultrasound scan would definitely be indicated to confirm the diagnosis of twins because twin pregnancies and twin births need special care and attention.

It can be quite a shock for a mother to be told that she is carrying twins and like any shock it can take a little time to get used to the idea. A very natural reaction is to deny that it's true. We've noticed a number of mothers have this experience. Our advice is that if you are told 'It's twins', take a little time to think about it yourself, then a little more time to talk about it with your husband or partner, then come back and talk to your midwife or your doctor or both. You are going to need special care during the pregnancy, and the birth.

Complications for Twins
Mothers carrying twins need extra attention because of the increased risk of anaemia, bleeding, polyhydramnios and pre-eclampsia.

Try to prevent anaemia by eating a good diet, just as for a single pregnancy. Get your blood count checked regularly (it should be done anyway) and take iron supplements if the count gets low (below 10g/l would be a guide most professionals would agree on). Bleeding in pregnancy always needs attention. Hydramnios and pre-eclampsia are discussed later in the book (see Chapters Four, Five and Six).

CHAPTER THREE

PLACE OF BIRTH

....

U ntil the recent publication of 'Changing Childbirth', the Government report on maternity services, it had not been widely realised
or understood that mothers could have any choice about where
they give birth. In fact, choice has always been possible, but we have to say
with some shame that professionals have attempted to conceal this
from mothers.

The choices available are at two levels. The first decision to make is
'Home or Hospital?'

In the first half of this century, home birth was commonplace, but since
the war, women have been increasingly encouraged to give birth in
hospital, to the extent that now only about one per cent of babies are born
at home. Nevertheless, over the last five years there has been a slow but
sure reversal of this trend. Women have, very reasonably, questioned
whether the practice of encouraging hospital births has led to real
improvements in care.

HOME OR HOSPITAL?

Evidence The pioneer researcher in this field was Marjorie Tew
who, in 1985, published an analysis of 17,972 births, the results of
which rocked the medical and midwifery world because her findings
suggested that the safest place to give birth was at home! There have
been arguments about this study ever since. The National Perinatal
Epidemiology Unit, based in Oxford, published a report in 1987

entitled 'Where to be born?: the debate and the evidence'. A second edition appeared in 1994. The first conclusion of these reports is 'There is no evidence to support the claim that the safest policy is for all women to give birth in hospital.'
Opinion We feel that for most women, birth at home is at least as safe as hospital birth.

There are advantages and disadvantages for both options:

Home

The advantages of home birth are a familiar environment with no restrictions on who can be present or not. The mother can be surrounded by people who love and care for her and attendants she knows and trusts. She can organise her own space with familiar, comfortable sights, sounds and smells. Relaxation is therefore easier to achieve at home.

We think that these factors lead to fewer complications in home births compared to hospital births. Results of an audit of home births in our practice confirm this is so. Mothers at home feel free to move about or to stay in one place, to eat and drink and adopt whatever position is comfortable. These are all factors which are known to ease the pain of labour. The absence of technology is an advantage for mothers at home. We find that our mothers who give birth at home are much less likely to have an episiotomy or a tear to the perineum than our mothers who give birth in hospital. It has been our experience, too, that involvement of the children of a family in the birth at home can be surprisingly positive. The fear of mothers is always that the children will be upset to see them distressed and in pain, but the distress seems to be much less in a home birth and we have attended many births in which the children were involved – sometimes very practically.

The disadvantages are that birth is messy (but in our case the doctor and midwife usually do most of the clearing up!) and some women undoubtedly feel more secure when surrounded by technology in hospital. If this is the case, then hospital is certainly the best place to be. Sadly for some women, even now, finding professional support for a home birth can be difficult. Epidural anaesthesia is not available at home, so if a mother wishes to use this technology, hospital is essential.

Many of our mothers have told us that they were regarded as being 'mad' by their friends when they said that they were going to have a home birth. Mothers seem to have been conditioned by doctors, and by society, to a belief that home birth is in some way unsafe or unsound. We do not believe that this conditioning has been a conscious or concerted plot on the part of the medical and midwifery professions. The doctors and obstetricians believed in good faith that by moving all births into hospital they would improve the chance of live healthy babies for all. This belief was even stated as government policy in the seventies. Consequently, since homebirth is now almost a rarity, many women fear that there is danger associated with homebirth. The **evidence** is that this is not so. 'What would happen if something goes wrong?' is the question our homebirth mothers are frequently asked by well-meaning but ill-informed friends. The answer to this is twofold: first, our experience and the statistics show that complications and emergencies are **less likely in a planned home birth**; secondly, when there is an emergency, midwives are fully competent to deal with any eventuality.

We carry all the equipment we would need to deal with any obstetric emergency. There is also the back-up of the ambulance service with trained paramedics at hand, ready to remove a mother and her baby to hospital quickly, if necessary, and also an Obstetric 'Flying Squad' for the emergency that requires action in the home itself. In our ten years of experience of increasing numbers of home births we have never had to use any of these facilities or the emergency equipment we carry! We have had to give resuscitation to only one baby, who merely required a little suction to his airway before he started breathing normally.

Vicki had her first baby in hospital, in the GP Unit. Her pregnancy was straightforward, and so was her labour and the birth, but as is often the case with first babies, her labour was long. She is an anxious person and found the hospital environment increased her anxiety. Changes of staff during her long labour increased the tension and sometimes she felt uncontrollably panicky. She now regards the experience in a very negative light. For her second baby, Vicki asked for a home birth. She was taught self-hypnosis to help control her feelings of panic. This time she had a much quicker labour, although this would be expected anyway for a second baby. She did not panic and felt in control the whole time, with two midwives she knew well attending her in her own home. She looks on this experience as a happy one. She says she can't stop talking about it.

Alice has five children, the last four of whom were born at home. We helped her with the last two of these. Alice suffered from post-natal depression after the third and fourth births and was frightened that this would happen again when she became pregnant for the fifth time. There were no problems during the pregnancy. Alice had the embarrassing experience of her waters breaking dramatically in a supermarket. Despite this, contractions did not start straight away, and after twenty-four hours, nothing had resulted. We then had a dilemma. There would be a risk of infection if labour did not start soon. Should Alice go to hospital for induction of labour with a syntocinon drip? She did not want to do this, so we started antibiotics as a precaution and waited.

The next morning, labour started properly. By mid-afternoon the contractions were very strong and Alice was finding them distressing. She wanted to know how she was progressing, so Kevan examined her, to find that the cervix had dilated to six centimetres. At this point, Alice became very distressed and said that she wanted to go to hospital and have an epidural. She could not stand the pain any more. Trish called the ambulance and rang the hospital to let them know we were coming. Meanwhile, Kevan talked to Alice to try to help her keep calm. As he was talking, he noticed that the baby's head was about to deliver! The baby, Finbar, was then born quite quickly, just before the ambulance arrived at the door to be turned away. Finbar did not breathe immediately, but after some suction to his airway, he was breathing normally and Alice was able to feed him. Three of Alice's children came in to watch when they knew that the baby was close. They did not get in the way, even when the little resuscitation was being carried out. Alice found them reassuring. When she said she wanted to go to hospital perhaps she was experiencing the fear which some think stimulates a response in the mother to give birth.

Hospital

The advantages of hospital birth are that some women feel more comfortable and secure there. If something should go wrong, they feel help is close at hand. Some feel safer when surrounded by technological equipment: electronic monitoring devices give some mothers a greater sense of security. There is a great deal of trust naturally felt for the local hospital, its midwives and medical staff. Someone else can deal with the mess. Perhaps being away from family and friends can be seen as an advantage. By far the majority of births take place in hospital now, and there may be a sense of complying with what most people do – what is socially acceptable. Epidural anaesthesia can be used to relieve pain. We will discuss the advantages and disadvantages of epidurals later.

The disadvantages of hospital birth are more restriction on movement, eating and drinking, and on who can be present. Although the theory is that getting up and walking about during labour is better for mothers, the central point of a hospital ward tends to be its beds. The bed is the place where mothers are expected to give birth and where they are expected to be for the greatest part of their time in labour. Electronic monitoring devices increase this restriction to the bed, literally tying mothers down. Hospital policies on eating and drinking in labour vary, but certainly one depends on the hospital kitchens for choice of food and drink. An unfamiliar environment leads to higher levels of anxiety. With the best of intentions from hospital staff, it is still recognised that there is a tendency to use technology even when it may not be appropriate or necessary.

Further Choices

In hospital there is a further level of choice between consultant care and GP care; some hospitals are also introducing midwife-led care. The consultant unit was originally intended as the place for complicated births but the trend has been for the majority of births to take place in such units. Since about 75% of births are normal births, this is an extreme solution which is also a waste of resources. It should be common sense that the specialists deal only with the complicated cases. If a mother has complications in pregnancy and needs consultant care, we think this should be available and that consultants should have the time free to spend with those who need them most. Conversely, GP or midwifery care is aimed at low-risk mothers and therefore tends to be less 'interventionist'. Provision of such units throughout the country, however, is sporadic. There has been a move towards closing GP units, especially those that are remote from the consultant units in large maternity hospitals, although these remote units have had excellent safety records. Midwifery units are a new departure, and hopefully their numbers will grow, but at present there are few, dealing with small numbers of cases.

Most GP or midwifery units are more relaxed and homely places in which to give birth. They are dedicated to 'normal' birth. There is great variety in the way GP units work. Some attached units have become integrated with the main hospital, so the consultants and GPs actually share a ward. Some occupy separate wings or floors of the hospital and some are in separate buildings on the same site. Policies for booking, and transfer of mothers to consultant care, also vary greatly, as does the amount of involvement of the local GPs.

For a small number of mothers there may be the opportunity to give birth in a 'birthing centre'. These are small units usually run by midwives in which they try to create the relaxed atmosphere of a home birth while having on hand facilities to deal with emergencies. Perhaps this will be increasingly available in the future.

Some more about GP Units

GP or midwifery units can be 'attached' to a District General Hospital or 'remote' – standing on their own, often at some distance from the main hospital. Both types can be run successfully and provide a good service to mothers. Geographical features often dictate which type of unit is found in which area – for example, free-standing units are found in more rural areas such as Brecon in south Wales and in Wiltshire and the Lake District. Attached units are more common in urban areas.

Not even the Department of Health knows how many GP units there are in the UK or where they are! So, unfortunately, we are unable to provide a list. There are several ways though that mothers can find out about GP units in their own area:

– other mothers may well be the best source of information, not only about where the units are located, but also about the kind of care offered and its quality;
– the NCT (National Childbirth Trust) local group will certainly know the local units;
– your Community Midwife probably works in one or more of the local units;
– your family doctor should have this information, but if the practice does not use the unit themselves, there may be some bias in the advice given. The same could equally be said on the other side if the practice are avid supporters of a local unit;
– if all else fails, the Community Health Council (CHC) will have good unbiased information. Their address and telephone number will be found in the local Directory. The CHC is a statutory body.

Negotiating your preferred choice

At your first visit, a good General Practitioner or midwife will:

– ask what you would like to happen about antenatal care and the place where you would like to give birth;
– discuss with you any potential problems that might arise in light of your medical history;
– explain what choices are open to you;
– arrive at an agreed plan of care for you and your baby.

It may be necessary at the first visit to perform some unintrusive examinations, such as feeling your tummy to check that the baby is about the right size for the dates you have worked out, or checking your blood pressure, but nothing else should be necessary at this stage.

The majority of family doctors and midwives will now adopt this approach, but we know from the letters and telephone calls we receive, that this is not always the case and that GPs are sometimes hostile to home birth, or midwifery-led care, so: **first ask for information about the choices open to you for your care**.

The doctor should be able to give you all the information you need to make choices about your care, but if you are not satisfied or feel that you have not been given an unbiased view, ask to see the community midwife.

The Department of Health have sent out a series of leaflets on choice in pregnancy aimed at helping women to make informed choices. These have been produced by Midirs and the NHS Centre for Reviews and Dissemination. They cover a number of topics including place of birth. They are aptly entitled 'Informed Choice for Women'. These should be available at the surgery or clinic. A similar series entitled 'Informed Choice for Professionals' covers the same topics for midwives and doctors. The leaflets are available directly from Midirs by telephoning 0891 210400 (calls costs 39p per minute off-peak, 49p at other times).

Take time to consider the information and make your choice. Pregnancy lasts for 40 weeks on average, so there should be no reason to hurry into a decision in the early months. Discuss what is on offer with your husband or partner and then ask for more information if you need it.

What to do if Not Satisfied with the Care Offered by your Family Doctor

1. Try to negotiate! It may be possible to come to some compromise about what you want; for example, a midwife may be able to provide your care during pregnancy, while you remain the patient of your own family doctor for all other medical problems.
2. Maternity Services are treated as separate from General Medical Services, and are paid for separately too. You do not have to get your maternity care from your family doctor. So if you can't reach an agreement, go elsewhere. You don't have to tell your GP you are doing this, but it may help good relations if you do. The District Health Authority will have a list of all the local GPs who provide maternity services and should also know which of them have a special interest in maternity care.
3. If all else fails, change your doctor.
4. If you can't find a GP anywhere to provide what you want, and you don't know a midwife, contact your local Midwifery Head of Maternity Services who should be based at the local maternity hospital. Ask her to provide you with a midwife who will give you all the care you need in pregnancy and birth. It is the duty of the Midwifery Head of Maternity Services to find you a midwife, so this is the bottom line! This approach should never fail.

We believe that the best care is provided by midwives and doctors working together. Each brings their own special knowledge and skills to the care of pregnant women. However, we regularly get phone calls and letters from women who are having difficulty with doctors! Our answer to them is always the same. Mothers-to-be do not need doctors for their care. The midwife is a skilled professional person, working with complete professional responsibility. If she needs the help of specialists, she has direct access to the consultant obstetricians at the local maternity hospital and she can order all the blood tests and scans that a mother might need in pregnancy.

If, as we hope, all goes well at the first visit to the doctor, the mother may be asked to come to an antenatal clinic run at the surgery, at which a midwife should be present. You may not have met the midwife before, so on your first visit, she may spend some time talking to you and finding out about your medical history, your family and your ideas about the care you would like. This meeting with the midwife may take place in your home.

Some GPs and midwives work together as we do, to provide care for most of the women in their community. Other doctors and midwives tend to refer most women to the local hospital for their care. At the hospital antenatal clinic, the same process of discussion and agreement about care should be provided. If it isn't, women should ask for it. Most women don't have much choice about which hospital to attend, but if you are lucky enough to have a choice, try to find out about the hospitals first. How is the antenatal clinic run? Is there a long wait at each visit or are women given appointments? What is the caesarean section rate in the hospital? What about the induction rate, episiotomy rate and facilities to encourage and support breast feeding? Your local NCT (National Childbirth Trust) group will probably have this information.

MORE ABOUT THE EVIDENCE

We think it's really important that mothers-to-be understand the evidence about place of birth, so at the risk of *labouring* it (sorry!), we'll summarise again what is known and consider some further evidence about psychological factors at birth.

Safety

There can now be no argument about the results of research which repeatedly show that **home birth is *at least* as safe as birth in hospital** for most women. Marjorie Tew (a statistician working at Nottingham University) analysed her very large number of births by classing each mother according to risk using criteria developed by obstetricians. The surprising results of her study were that in each risk group, even in the highest risk pregnancies, the outcome was better for home births than for hospital births. Further analyses and studies by the National Perinatal Epidemiology Unit have confirmed that at the least, there is no difference between home and hospital in terms of outcome. Recently, a prospective survey was carried out in the northern region of England with two aims: to assess safety by looking at the outcome of pregnancy, and to test the availability of choice and satisfaction of women wanting a home birth. There were no perinatal deaths in 139 home births in the region in 1993 (perinatal mortality 0.0). The perinatal mortality for the region in the same year, which in practice represents the rate for the hospitals in the region, was 9.1 per thousand.

Choice

'Changing Childbirth', the 1994 Government report on maternity care, states that women should receive unbiased information in order to be able to choose the place of birth, and that real choice should be made available to women. In practice, choice is still limited, as we know from the letters and phone calls we get from women. In the Northern Regional Home-birth Survey, only nine mothers asking for home birth had a GP who was supportive. 65% of mothers in the survey said that they were not given any choice about place of birth by their GPs. We think it is likely that similar problems also apply to women choosing a GP unit or Midwifery unit birth but perhaps to a lesser extent. Despite this depressing evidence, we believe that women themselves can bring about change and take the choice that is being withheld from them. To do this, mothers should remember two points which we'll recap:

– a doctor is not necessary for a birth in any setting. The midwife is fully competent to manage all aspects of normal birth and antenatal care, and to refer to specialist help when needed. To choose a homebirth or a Midwifery unit birth, a mother does **not** need the permission or presence of her doctor;
– Maternity Medical Services are provided separately from General Medical Services and a woman is free to choose a GP different from her own for her maternity care.

Wendy, like Vicki, is an anxious person and felt that her anxiety was made worse by the two births she had in hospital. For the third she decided to have a home birth. Jenny was born at home after a short labour, at three in the morning. She was obviously a Downs baby. We decided not to tell her parents immediately after the birth, but left it until we came back in daylight. They had realised themselves by then, but say that they were very grateful to us for allowing them a few hours of happiness and peace before breaking bad news.

Two years later Wendy decided to have another baby. She had screening, a detailed ultrasound scan and amniofiltration (a method similar to amniocentesis which was the subject of research, but has now been abandoned), all of which showed that this was a normal baby. She was determined that she wanted to have the baby at home. During the pregnancy Wendy came under enormous pressure to have a hospital birth from various people including the paediatrician who was looking after Jenny, a psychologist and other professionals with whom she came into contact. These people gave unsolicited advice when they were not responsible for Wendy's maternity care, and nor were they experts in the field. The advice they gave was illogical because the risk involved in a hospital birth is, as we have shown, at least the same as for a home birth, and the risk of Downs' syndrome is unaffected by place of birth. Further, we knew already that the baby did not have a chromosome abnormality. Wendy resisted this pressure and Richard was born without complication, at home, in water. It was a few days before Christmas and the tree in the room gave the event an extra beauty.

Satisfaction with Birth

The 'Changing Childbirth' report recognised that the mother's feelings about birth and her satisfaction with the way in which she gives birth are important, and that safety, although of first importance, is not the only factor that should be considered in decisions about place of birth. The report says: 'Safety is not an absolute concept. It is part of a greater picture encompassing all aspects of health and well-being.'

The Northern Homebirth Survey identified some of the factors that women felt were important in choosing a home birth. These were:

- Feeling more in control
- Being more relaxed
- More natural
- Partner more involved
- Less intervention
- Less stress for baby
- Not having to leave the other children
- Privacy
- Safety

Some of these ideas could also relate to hospital birth. When women who had given birth in hospital before were asked about their preference, 85% preferred the home birth, even though many of these found the hospital experience satisfactory. 34% said that their hospital experience had been unpleasant, impersonal and that they had dealt with a lot of different people, that there were interventions that they felt to be unnecessary, and that there was a lack of sleep and of privacy.

Carol's Story

Carol, at 36, was the mother of one little girl. She was now pregnant again and wrote to us asking if we would look after her for a home birth. She wished to use a birthing pool. She had approached her own doctor who had refused. As she lived outside our area, some distance from the practice, we felt there would be difficulties for us in helping her but gave our standard response in such situations. We advised Carol that she did not need a doctor to look after her in pregnancy or during labour and that she should be able to find a midwife in her own area who would care for her.

Another month went by. Carol rang up saying that she had approached the midwife attached to her GP's practice, but that she was not willing to give the care she wanted. We advised Carol to contact her local director of midwives. After another month we received another letter from Carol. She had done as we suggested, and the director of midwives had put her in touch with a local group of midwives. These midwives worked as a team (this is a trend called team midwifery which has its advantages and disadvantages) and although some members of the team were comfortable with a water birth at home, others were not. Carol felt that if she were to go into labour at the wrong time, according to the midwives' rota, she could end up in hospital for the birth; she was keen not to do this unless there was some pressing reason.

At this point we gave up and decided to look after Carol on the understanding that if there were any difficulties about the distance taking us away from our own patients, she would go in to the local GP unit and use our birthing pool there. In the event Carol's blood pressure went up to a high level at the end of a previously uncomplicated pregnancy and she required transfer to consultant care and induction. She gave birth to a little girl, weighing 7lb 4oz, in the pool. She had no need for stitches and had no further complications.

Carol's story illustrates several difficulties for mothers wanting home birth or indeed any deviation from the routine of hospital birth. Her doctor had no experience of home birth and certainly none of water birth.

It was only reasonable that she could not help, but this left the midwife attached to the practice in an uncomfortable position. A midwife in this situation should have full professional responsibility and autonomy. Team midwifery has its advantages for midwives in terms of getting time off but unless all the members of a team are of one mind and equally experienced, then the mothers may be disadvantaged because of conflicting advice or the luck of the draw with a rota. Unless the team is very small, the mother may still find she is being looked after in labour by a midwife she has never met before.

Checklist for Local Maternity Hospital

Antenatal Care:
- Can this be shared with local GP or midwife?
- Do antenatal clinics have an appointment system?
- How many appointments are given during a clinic?
- Is it possible to see the consultant responsible for care?
- Is it possible to have midwifery-led care?

Birth:
- Is there a GP or Midwifery unit?
- How can a booking into such a unit be arranged?
- Is there a 'low technology unit'?
- Is epidural analgesia available?
- What is the caesarean section rate?
- What is the induction rate?
- What is the episiotomy rate?

Postnatal Care:
- What support is available for breast-feeding?
- What is the usual length of stay in hospital after the birth?

Decision Chart for Place of Birth

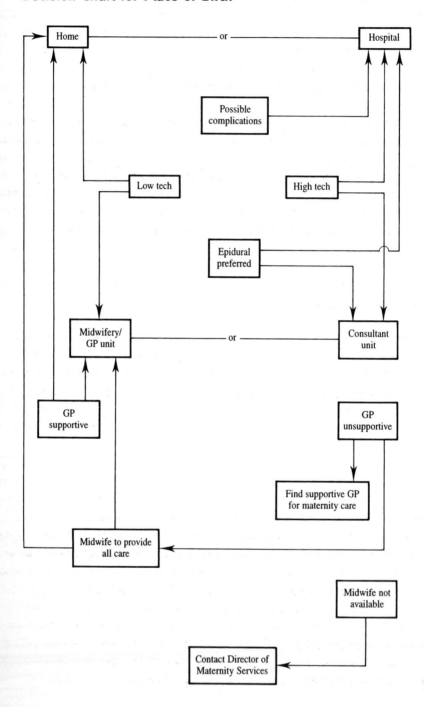

C H A P T E R F O U R

IS OUR BABY NORMAL? – SCREENING

....

What is screening?

The idea of screening is simple; if disease can be detected at an early stage then treatment may be more effective. Better still, if those *at risk of developing a disease* can be identified and treated, then the disease can be prevented altogether. So to put it simply, the idea of screening is to use some sort of test to try to identify disease early, and to find people '*at risk*' of getting a disease.

'Pros and Cons' of Screening

If this concept is applied to maternity care, then antenatal care can be seen as a form of screening. The objectives of screening in pregnancy are twofold – to prevent disease in the mother and to ensure, as far as is possible, a healthy baby. These sound like excellent aims, and screening certainly contributes to the health of mother and baby, but unfortunately life is rarely simple and straightforward and there are disadvantages of screening as well as advantages. In our experience the 'pros and cons' of screening are rarely put to mothers. Mothers are often told things like 'You should have this test to make sure the baby is all right.' We believe that it is important for mothers to understand the benefits and risks of screening before committing themselves to tests. For example, ultrasound scanning is widely used in antenatal care, and is, as far as we can tell, safe, but what are the long-term results? We'll discuss this in detail later.

TIP

Before agreeing to any tests, make sure you understand the risks and benefits involved.

Think it through

It is a good idea to have thought through the consequences of a positive result of a test – '*What shall we do if something is wrong?*'

For example, in screening for Downs' syndrome if there was a positive result:

– Would we carry on with the pregnancy come what may, knowing that there is a chance that the baby may be handicapped in some way?
– Or do we want to know for certain whether there is an abnormality or not, even though the tests that will give us this diagnosis may increase the chance of miscarriage.
– Will we consider 'terminating' the pregnancy by having an abortion if we know there is a risk of handicap?
– Or do we want to know about the risk of handicap, even though we would never consider an abortion, so that we can prepare for the possibility of a handicapped child.

Hidden screening

Some screening procedures are performed routinely in antenatal clinics without much thought either by the professionals or the mothers. Below is a list of screening tests which most mothers will be offered during pregnancy. Some of these are not always thought of as screening and may cause surprise. Most doctors agree that screening is not appropriate when there is no adequate treatment for the disease or problem being screened for. This raises difficult questions for both mother and professionals when it is the baby who is being screened and the only 'treatment' available is to terminate the pregnancy by inducing abortion.

SCREENING TESTS FOR THE MOTHER

Screening Test	Disease/Problem looked for	Treatment
Blood pressure measurement	Pre-eclampsia	Bed rest and possibly early delivery Sometimes antihypertensive drugs
Urine testing	Diabetes Urinary tract infection Pre-eclampsia	Diet or medication Antibiotics See above
Abdominal palpation (feeling the tummy)	Fetal growth retardation	None
Auscultation of the fetal heart (Listening)	Fetal death	None
Blood samples for haemoglobin	Anaemia	Iron or blood transfusion

SCREENING TESTS FOR THE BABY

Screening Test	Disease/Problem looked for	Treatment
Blood groups	Haemolytic disease of the newborn	Rhesus immunisation
Blood tests for sexually transmitted disease	Congenital STD in the newborn	Antibiotics
Ultrasound scanning	Fetal abnormality	Termination of pregnancy
	Poor fetal growth	None
	Placenta praevia	Possibly caesarean section
AFP (alpha-fetoprotein) Double, triple or triple-plus marker tests	Downs syndrome and spina bifida	Termination of pregnancy

Getting information about screening

Recent surveys of women in antenatal care have shown that most women do not actually know what tests they have had. Nor do they know what the tests were for. This cannot be the fault of the women; rather, a failure of communication on the part of professionals.

We believe that it is wrong to perform any of these screening tests routinely without adequate explanation to mothers about the test itself, its safety and the possible consequences of a positive result. We try to give information to mothers in our antenatal clinic groups and encourage them to discuss these issues among themselves. When this facility is not available, it is important for mothers to ask the doctors or midwives for information about any tests they are offered. Don't be satisfied with 'It's to make sure your baby is all right'. This is not a logical statement because the implication is 'this procedure will confirm that your baby is healthy', which is of course what most mothers want to hear. The very nature of a screening test is that statistically most mothers will be told that the baby is healthy, but what if the test is positive? Having the test in this case will **not** make sure that the baby is all right! Treatment is available for only a tiny number of abnormalities that can be detected by screening, and often the only 'treatment' that can be offered is termination of pregnancy. To terminate a pregnancy is a very difficult decision for any mother to make. Equally, it is extremely hard for a mother to continue with a pregnancy in the knowledge that she is carrying an abnormal baby, taking into account the future consequences for the child's life.

This makes decisions about whether to have screening tests very complex, but our experience is that mothers prefer to have thought through these problems and to make their choices based on information. Some women decide when given this information that they would rather not know, and decline the tests. Others decide that in no circumstances could they bear the consequences of delivering a child with a handicap or abnormality. Both positions should be respected by midwives and doctors and no one should be made to feel guilty about decisions they have made either to have or not to have the tests.

Screening and Diagnosis

It is important to understand the difference between screening and diagnosis. A screening test is used to detect *possible* cases of a disease or to identify people *at risk*. It does **not** confirm that any individual person has the disease. Diagnosis means finding a specific disease in a particular person.

An example is the AFP test for Downs' syndrome. A positive result (a low level of alpha feto-protein in the mother's blood) does not necessarily mean that the baby has Downs' syndrome. It does indicate an *increased risk* of Downs' syndrome for that mother. It is possible to put an estimate of risk against the result and most centres performing the tests now express the results in terms of risk. A mother might therefore be told 'your risk is one in 400 – that means 399 to one, your baby does *not* have Downs' syndrome on the basis of this test'. Doctors choose, arbitrarily, a cut-off point for the risk of Downs' syndrome, below which the test is regarded as positive. In most centres this would be one in 250. So the test is regarded as positive and the mother offered further investigation if the risk is worse than that figure.

Diagnosis can only be made by amniocentesis or some similar procedure. This involves inserting a needle into the womb, withdrawing fluid from around the baby and culturing the cells in the fluid to see whether the baby has the abnormal chromosomes that cause Downs' syndrome. This test gives an almost certain answer to the question 'does my baby have Downs' syndrome?' – either yes or no within the limits of laboratory error (which is very unusual). However, the amniocentesis test is not without risk to the baby.

Limitations of Screening

There seems to be a belief, which has been cultivated partly by the medical profession and partly by the media, that it is possible to detect, and therefore eradicate, almost every abnormality in unborn babies. Nothing could be further from the truth. Only a small number of possible abnormalities can be detected by screening in pregnancy. There are no tests for the vast majority of disabling conditions. Further, even the screening tests that are available do not detect every case. Two-thirds of all babies with Downs' syndrome are born to women who were not considered to be at risk.

Some more about the Tests

Let's consider each of the tests in the list above and weigh up the various 'pros and cons'.

Blood Pressure

High blood pressure in pregnancy is not in itself a problem for mother or baby, but a rise in blood pressure does indicate an increase in risk. High blood pressure, with *proteinuria* (protein in the urine), means a serious condition known as pre-eclampsia or pre-eclamptic toxaemia (which is now an old-fashioned term). This condition is important and does give substantial risks to mother and baby. Increased blood pressure on its own is quite common in pregnancy, and indeed it is normal for the blood pressure to go up a little during the first three months, fall during the middle three months and increase again towards the end of pregnancy. Pre-eclampsia, on the other hand, is relatively uncommon, but potentially very serious.

No one knows when their blood pressure is high. There are no signs or symptoms. So although the disease (pre-eclampsia) for which we are looking is relatively uncommon compared to the number of normal results from blood pressure checks in antenatal clinics, the consequences of pre-eclampsia are so serious that checking blood pressure must remain an important part of antenatal care. What is uncertain is how often it is necessary to check the blood pressure in a pregnancy.

Logically the beginning and end are important times, but how often in-between is still a matter of debate. Some researchers have found that five antenatal check-ups, at booking, 16 weeks, 26 weeks, 30 weeks, 36 weeks and full term, are all that is necessary for good antenatal care. The blood pressure is checked on each of these occasions. On the other hand, some doctors with a special interest in blood pressure have argued that this number of check-ups may be insufficient to pick up the dangerous condition of high blood pressure arising during the middle period of pregnancy.

At present, there is **no evidence** to support either view but we find, from our experience, that a smaller number of antenatal check-ups is better, and we feel that we should give mothers the right of access to antenatal care when they feel it is needed. We think that mothers are likely to know when something is wrong and feel strongly that when a mother comes to a doctor or midwife, and says that she feels something is wrong, even if she cannot be sure exactly what it is, then this intuitive feeling should be taken very seriously indeed. We think this intuition also applies to blood-pressure checking.

Safety: Taking someone's blood pressure may seem to be a harmless procedure, but there are hidden risks involved in taking the blood pressure too often. Research has shown that everyone's blood pressure tends to go up when they attend a hospital or a doctor's surgery. This certainly applies in antenatal clinics no matter how relaxed they are, and many are far from relaxed. Mothers' blood pressure is known to be higher in clinics than if it is taken at home. Mothers with 'high' blood pressure are more likely to be given induction of labour and therefore more intervention in labour, including a higher risk of caesarean section. This is true even though it is known that a rise of blood pressure **alone** at the end of pregnancy does not give a worse outcome for mother or baby. Taking the blood pressure is therefore like any other screening test. There is a risk associated with false positive results.

Urine testing

Urine is tested for sugar and protein. Testing for protein is important because of pre-eclampsia (see above). Proteinuria may also indicate urinary tract infection which often occurs without symptoms in pregnancy. Three to eight per cent of pregnant women have bacteriuria (infection by bacteria in the urine) without symptoms – they don't know they've got it. 15% to 45% of women with symptomless bacteriuria will get cystitis or pyelonephritis (infections of the bladder or kidneys) unless they are treated. Testing the urine for sugar is important in order to detect diabetes, since the outcome of pregnancy is worse for diabetics, especially if uncontrolled. There is a threefold increase in the risk of fetal abnormalities for diabetic mothers. Diabetic mothers tend to have larger babies and if the mother has kidney problems, high blood pressure in pregnancy may make these worse. Again there is no research evidence which indicates how often the urine should be tested in pregnancy. We feel that it is probably unnecessary to test at every visit unless there is some indication to do so, such as the woman's past medical history or a previous positive test.

Abdominal palpation

This means feeling the tummy. There are various reasons for performing this examination but for the greater part of pregnancy its purpose is to check on the growth of the baby. It is a fairly imprecise test, relying on the experience of the examiner to assess normality. Increasingly, tape measures are used to measure the symphysio-fundal height (the distance between the top of the uterus and the pubic bone of the mother's pelvis, both of which can be felt through the abdomen).

TAPE MEASURING

Evidence This would seem logically to be a more accurate assessment of growth but research indicates that it is no more accurate than simple palpation. Further research is still needed in this area.

Towards the end of pregnancy, palpation gives important information about the way the baby is lying which has consequences for the birth.

Abdominal palpation is a safe procedure, but done by the inexperienced or insensitive it can cause considerable discomfort for mothers. Our advice is if someone causes you discomfort, **tell them**.

Listening to the fetal heart

It is very reassuring for mothers and professionals to know that the baby's heart is beating.

AUSCULTATION

Evidence This test is more accurate when the doppler machine or 'sonicaid' is used instead of the old-fashioned ear trumpet. The sonicaid also has the advantage that the mother (and anyone else in the room) can hear the heartbeat too. The heart can be heard as early as 16 weeks with the sonicaid. Of course if the heartbeat cannot be heard this is very serious and may mean that the baby has died, in which case no action is possible, but such tragedies are becoming increasingly rare. The reassurance for the vast majority of mothers hearing for themselves that all is well must outweigh the very rare disasters.

Safety: The old ear trumpet, known as the 'Pinard's' stethoscope, is perfectly safe. So too probably is the sonicaid, but what many mothers probably do not realise is that this machine does use doppler ultrasound. The 'dose' of ultrasound given to the baby each time the machine is used is very small but perhaps these exposures of the baby to ultrasound are additive. Not enough research has been done to check this.

Blood tests for haemoglobin

Haemoglobin, the red pigment in blood cells, falls normally in pregnancy because of dilution of the blood.

FALLING HAEMOGLOBIN

Evidence This normal process is associated with a better outcome than when the haemoglobin is artificially raised to 'normal' non-pregnant levels by giving iron supplements. Despite the evidence, doctors and midwives often seem to be obsessed with levels of haemoglobin and may rush to treat 'low' levels inappropriately. There are many side effects of iron including bowel disturbance – constipation or diarrhoea – which are particularly unpleasant for expectant mothers. There is some evidence of a possible teratogenic effect of iron (it might cause fetal abnormalities) but the risk of this would be very small.

It is not the haemoglobin level that should be treated but the mother and her baby! Perhaps the reason for the desire to give treatment for apparent anaemia, is that tiredness is a common symptom of pregnancy. Doctors, midwives and mothers may therefore put two and two together and make five (or 9.5 in the case of haemoglobin), attributing this tiredness to low haemoglobin. Both professionals and mothers forget that the haemoglobin level is a screening test. Like all such tests it does not give a diagnosis. To make a diagnosis of anaemia, the other 'indices' or measurements of constituents of the blood must be taken into consideration. Only genuine iron-deficiency anaemia should be treated with iron supplements. There is no evidence that tiredness in pregnancy can be reduced by iron supplements.

Blood Groups

There is no doubt that the understanding of rhesus blood group incompatibility and immunisation for mothers to prevent rhesus incompatibility represents one of the most important advances in medical science in the twentieth century, which has resulted in the saving of many babies' lives and the prevention of serious illness in many others. The procedures involved are safe and effective.

Haemolytic disease of the newborn is caused by a rhesus negative mother carrying a rhesus positive baby; the baby's blood cells are destroyed by antibodies to rhesus positive cells in the mother's blood. The antibodies will only be present if there has been previous sensitisation of the mother by red blood cells from a baby carrying rhesus antigens (a rhesus positive baby). This sensitisation occurs most often at the birth of a first child, when blood from the placenta releases red cells from the baby into the mother's circulation. The antibodies which result from this reaction can cross the placenta in the next pregnancy and attack the baby's blood cells.

Not every baby with rhesus incompatibility (rhesus negative mother, rhesus positive baby) would be affected by these antibodies. In fact, the risk if no treatment were available would be about one in 170. This is because leakage of the baby's blood into the mother's circulation does not always occur in sufficient quantity to produce sensitisation and some women do not produce antibodies even if there is a large leakage. If the father has genes for rhesus negative and rhesus positive blood, he will be rhesus positive, but the baby has a 50% chance of being positive or negative. Finally, in about 20% of potential cases, antibody production is prevented by interaction with the other blood group systems. In other words, the baby's red cells that leak into the mother are destroyed if their ABO group is different from that of the mother and so no rhesus antibodies are produced.

Rhesus haemolytic disease is now very rare, mainly because of immunisation of rhesus negative mothers after birth. This is done by giving antirhesus antibody to rhesus negative mothers immediately after a birth or a miscarriage. This destroys any rhesus positive cells in the mother's circulation before they have time to do any harm. This treatment has been shown to be safe and effective in a number of research studies in different countries. The immunisation is known as anti-D. There are other rhesus blood groups known as Kell, Kidd and Duffy after their discoverers. These very rarely cause problems but most hospital laboratories test the blood of mothers routinely for them.

A natural fall in the number of cases of rhesus haemolytic disease has also resulted from the reduction in family size during the second half of the century, because first babies are not affected by the condition.

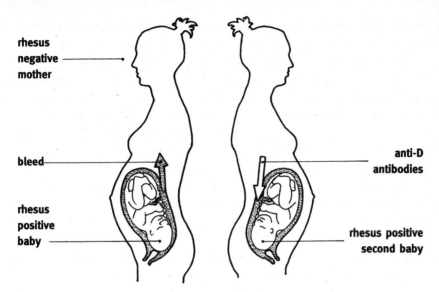

rhesus negative mother

bleed

rhesus positive baby

anti-D antibodies

rhesus positive second baby

Sensitisation of rhesus negative mother by bleed leading to the production of anti-D antibodies.

The rhesus positive blood cells in the second baby are affected by antibodies crossing the placenta.

Testing for sexually transmitted disease

It is probably a surprise to most mothers to hear that in the majority of hospitals they would be routinely tested for syphilis by taking a blood sample. Although a rare condition, the consequences for the baby from catching the disease from an infected mother are potentially disastrous and treatment with antibiotics is effective. There remains controversy about routine screening for other sexually transmitted diseases and particularly HIV. At present, routine HIV testing is **not** carried out in British hospitals.

Ultrasound scanning

Scanning can be used in screening to check the gestational age of the baby, to detect fetal abnormalities, to check for poor growth of the baby and to check the site of the placenta. The scanner works by sending high frequency sound waves into the mother's body and detecting the reflections from the baby. These reflections are then converted into a two-dimensional picture by computerised wizardry.

Indications for scanning

Early pregnancy: Scans can be used to check the gestational age of the baby when the mother is unsure of the dates or there is inconsistency between the mother's dates and the size of the baby. Ultrasound can also be useful in detecting twins or other multiples. If there are clinical signs of an ectopic pregnancy (one outside the uterus), scanning will confirm the diagnosis.

Anomaly scanning: The optimum time for checking for fetal abnormalities, such as Downs syndrome or other problems, is 20 weeks, but many departments combine the anomaly scan with a scan for 'dates' at 16 weeks, to coincide with the blood test for AFP (see later).

Late Pregnancy: Scans can be used to check the site of the placenta (afterbirth) when Placenta praevia is suspected. They are also used to check on the growth of the baby – and this is probably when they are least accurate.

Mother's Request: Because we do our own scanning, we get quite a few requests from mothers for scans for various reasons including wanting the father to see the baby, wanting to know the sex of the baby, wanting a photograph or just for reassurance. We would suggest that mothers think carefully before asking for a scan for such reasons and consider the risks as well as the benefits.

Routine versus indicated scanning

We find that most of our mothers now expect to have a scan as a matter of routine. They seem to have been conditioned to this view by the experience of their friends and by the media, and probably by the attitude of professionals. Most hospitals now seem to perform scanning as a routine, and most give women a minimum of two scans – an early scan for dating and a late scan at 30 or 32 weeks) for placental site and to check growth. Some do more scanning as routine. This is surprising as there is no evidence of its value.

ROUTINE SCANNING

Evidence Late pregnancy ultrasound has been shown by research studies to be inaccurate at diagnosing growth retardation. In particular, the writers of *Effective Care in Pregnancy and Childbirth*, which is a book based on the research evidence collated by the National Perinatal Epidemiology Centre, conclude that the research evidence available does not support the use of routine ultrasound in late pregnancy. They consider that routine use of ultrasound in early pregnancy should be balanced against possible risks, since safety is unproven.

There is no argument either from research evidence collected or among doctors and midwives about the value of diagnostic ultrasound used **for specific indications**.

Transvaginal ultrasound

This means a probe being inserted into the vagina so that ultrasound signals can reach the baby without having first to pass through the mother's abdominal wall. The vaginal probe gets much nearer to the baby than the abdominal probe, so the power of the ultrasound is higher. This gives higher resolution and is therefore particularly effective in very early pregnancy. It is used commonly in infertility clinics. There is a small risk of infection associated with the use of vaginal ultrasound, which is obviously an invasive and intrusive procedure for the woman. The safety of the procedure for the baby has not been studied, but this procedure will be used in pregnancy, at a time when the baby is developing all its organs. The potential for harm is greater because of the probable increase in the 'dose' of ultrasound received by the baby and the time of development at which the equipment is used.

Doppler ultrasound

This is being increasingly used in special centres where its main indication is in checking the blood flow through the uterine arteries which provide the blood supply to the womb and therefore to the baby. Potentially this technique would give a more accurate diagnosis of intra-uterine growth retardation (IUGR) and might eventually lead to the development of treatment for this condition, but at present there is no treatment.

Safety: Scanning has been used for over 30 years without any reports of serious harm to the babies. There are, however, concerns about the use of scanning, especially 'routine' scanning in pregnancy.

SCANNING AND SAFETY

Evidence There have been studies showing an association between frequent scans in pregnancy and the development of dyslexia in children. There have also been studies in animals showing damage to cells caused by ultrasound at the levels used in obstetrics and some scientists have expressed concern about the possible effects on future generations of scanning carried out now. No large studies of the safety of scanning have been carried out and although there is little evidence of harm from scanning, like many technologies, there is a temptation to use it without thinking. This is especially true of ultrasound because it is apparently so safe and there is the bonus to the mother of seeing her baby on the screen, and even taking away a picture. There is certainly **no evidence** that the **routine** use of ultrasound in pregnancy improves the outcome for mother or baby. The World Health Organisation has expressed concern about such routine use.

The 'dose' of ultrasound that the baby receives from scanning may be important. It is quite difficult to calculate the dose received, and indeed, the baby receives ultrasound waves from sources other than scans, for example, the sonicaid used to listen to the fetal heart and the electronic monitor used in labour. No one knows whether the effects of all this exposure are additive.

Scanning is never 100% accurate, and there have been recent reports of women being advised to have abortions on the basis of a scan showing some abnormality when in fact the baby was completely normal. Tragically, these discoveries were made by post-mortem examinations of the aborted babies.

A tragic case was brought to the attention of AIMS (The Association for Improvement in Maternity Services). A midwife was looking after a young woman who mentioned worries about her second pregnancy because her first baby had been aborted due to hydrocephalus (a condition of too much fluid surrounding the brain which can result in brain damage). This was found by ultrasound scanning. When the midwife looked at the case notes, she found that the post-mortem revealed no abnormality. The mother had not been told this result! When the midwife told her, she accepted the tragedy as an error of judgement but was relieved that her present baby was not damaged.

Use of ultrasound in screening for fetal abnormalities
Women who wish to have AFP testing or screening for Downs' syndrome by markers in maternal blood, will certainly need a scan to determine gestational age accurately. This is because the levels of markers used for Downs' screening vary with gestational age.

Ultrasound in itself, in the hands of experienced sonographers, can be a useful screening test for Downs' syndrome and for other abnormalities. It can be very reassuring to know that all is well with the baby, but before allowing herself to be scanned for abnormalities, we would advise a mother to think carefully about the consequences of an abnormal result. What will parents do with the knowledge that their baby may be handicapped in some way? It must be remembered that scanning cannot provide an absolute diagnosis, only a suggestion that something *may* be wrong.

Most sonographers agree that the best time to scan for abnormalities is 20 weeks. By this time the baby is quite large. Termination of pregnancy, which in the vast majority of cases is the only form of treatment available for an abnormality detected, is more unpleasant physically and emotionally than in early pregnancy. Many women who decide that in no circumstances would they entertain termination of pregnancy, may feel that it would be better not to be screened. Others may feel that they could not give birth to a handicapped child under any circumstances. For them the uncertainty of screening by scanning may provide insufficient information on which to make a decision. We should all, mothers, doctors and midwives, try to avoid the disaster of mothers being given wrong advice on the basis of ultrasound, and normal pregnancies being terminated.

SCANNING – OUR CONCLUSIONS

Opinion Ultrasound scanning can give useful information which is helpful in the management of pregnancy when there is a clinical indication for its use. Sometimes it can be lifesaving for the baby, but there is no evidence to support routine use of ultrasound in pregnancy and its safety has not been proven.

We would like to see doctors, midwives and mothers all think more about the indications for scanning. We advise our mothers whenever they are offered a scan (even by ourselves) to ask what the purpose of it is and not to be satisfied with that glib answer 'it's to check that the baby is all right.'

Ultrasound Checklist

- ◆ Is my scan for a particular reason or just routine?
- ◆ Have the reasons been explained clearly?

- Is there a less risky way of obtaining the information to be found by the scan?
- What sort of ultrasound will be used?
- How long will the baby be exposed to the ultrasound?
- How many scans do I need?
- How can I minimise the 'dose' of ultrasound given to the baby?

Screening for Downs' syndrome and other fetal abnormalities by testing mothers' blood

Alpha-fetoprotein is a substance produced by the baby which is found in the mother's blood. Low levels are associated with a higher risk of the baby having Downs' syndrome, higher levels with spina bifida and other 'neural tube defects'. Other chemical substances or cells in the blood, known as 'markers', have been used in the tests and the addition of each marker improves the power of the test to detect an abnormality. Most regions now offer the mother a two-marker test. Some use a 'triple test' and in Leeds there is a 'triple plus' test with four markers. This test is available to every mother in the country by payment of a fee of approximately £100. St James's University Hospital in Leeds provides an excellent advice and counselling service with this test. For further information, contact The Medical Coordinator, Downs' Syndrome Screening Service, Department of Obstetrics and Gynaecology, St James's University Hospital, Leeds LS9 7TF (01532 344013).

It is very important for mothers and fathers to understand the purpose and limitations of these screening tests **before** agreeing to have them. These tests do **not** give a diagnosis. A risk estimate can be calculated from the results of the test and the decision as to whether a test is positive or negative is based on this risk estimate. The level of risk which is considered acceptable is arbitrary and has been chosen by doctors. In most regions the 'cut-off point' is a risk of one in 250 that the baby has Downs' syndrome. Many people would consider this a pretty remote chance. The diagnosis of Downs' syndrome in a baby can only be made by an invasive technique such as amniocentesis. This carries its own risks – one per cent of women undergoing amniocentesis will miscarry. No one expects to have a positive result from screening but when a mother is faced with the news that her screening test was positive (ie there might be something wrong with the baby), it can lead to great distress and confusion. For this reason, it is a good idea to have thought out beforehand what action you would take if you got a positive result.

Karen had the terrible experience of being told that her AFP test was positive (with a risk of one in 240). She had chosen a consultant unit booking and was told the result when she attended the antenatal clinic. She says, 'I thought it was very badly handled. I got the impression he (the consultant) thought I already knew. I felt very much abandoned. I think a lot of people have the tests without really thinking it through.' Although Karen's risk was really quite low, her husband felt that he could not cope with the thought that there might be something wrong, so Karen decided to have amniocentesis. She says, 'Everyone was very nice on the actual day and the amniocentesis was fine, but I discovered when I got the result that they'd had it for two weeks. I was worried for four weeks and it's a long time to wait. It's not something I'd like to repeat.' Karen's amniocentesis showed that the baby had normal karyotype, which means she did not have Downs' syndrome. Her baby was born normally five months later.

Diagnosis of Downs' syndrome

In order to make a diagnosis of Downs' syndrome, or any other rarer chromosome abnormality during pregnancy, it is necessary to perform some sort of invasive procedure. Amniocentesis is the older method, which has been used and refined over some 20 years. Chorionic villus sampling (CVS) is a more recently developed technique. Other methods are the subject of research but all have one thing in common: a needle must be inserted into the uterus, usually through the mother's abdomen, and a sample withdrawn from the fluid surrounding the baby, or from the chorionic trophoblast which is the early placenta. These methods are *diagnostic* which means that they tell with as near to certainty as one can in medicine (nothing is ever 100%) whether the baby has a chromosome defect or not.

TIP

Remember: these methods only diagnose chromosome defects; there can be no certainty that a baby is completely 'normal' even with a negative (good) result.

Amniocentesis

This is a technique for diagnosing chromosome abnormalities, the most common by far being Downs' syndrome. It is done between 14 and 20 weeks of pregnancy by inserting a needle through the abdominal wall of the mother, into the uterus and into the fluid surrounding the baby (the amniotic fluid). A sample is withdrawn and sent for cell culture. The procedure should be done under ultrasound control so that the doctor can see the baby and the needle. The fluid contains cells from the baby which can be cultured in a laboratory so that the chromosomes can be examined. We all have 46 chromosomes (23 pairs). Downs' babies have an extra chromosome, number 21. There are some rarer abnormalities in which chromosomes or parts of chromosomes are missing, or there are extra chromosomes of a different number. 'Trisomy' – meaning three chromosomes – of the 14–15 and 16–18 groups causes mental handicap. A missing part of chromosome number 5 causes the 'cri du chat' syndrome in which the baby has cystic fibrosis and a strange mewing cry. Two conditions caused by abnormal sex chromosomes are 'Klinefelter's syndrome' in which there is an additional X-chromosome. People with this condition are often not recognised because despite often having mixed (male and female) secondary sexual characteristics, they look like 'normal' males. Turner's syndrome is caused by a missing X-chromosome and results in a female with a characteristic short webbed neck. These people may be infertile.

Risks of amniocentesis
The disadvantage of this procedure is that one per cent of mothers who undergo amniocentesis will miscarry. This statistic applies when the procedure is done by an experienced doctor. In inexperienced hands, the miscarriage rate is even higher. If performed later in pregnancy, the complications of termination of pregnancy are greater than earlier on.

Chorionic Villus Sampling (CVS)
This can be done earlier than amniocentesis, from nine to 14 weeks. CVS is done by inserting a needle either through the abdomen, or via the vagina into the uterus, again under ultrasound control, and removing a small piece of trophoblast tissue (early placenta) to examine the cells for chromosome abnormalities. It was hoped that this procedure, performed earlier, would have advantages over amniocentesis because of the earlier stage of pregnancy at which a termination could be made following a positive result. However, the miscarriage rate is about the same as for amniocentesis, and it has been found that if performed between eight and 11 weeks, there is a risk of damage to the limbs of the baby, so some of the advantage has been lost.

Jane and Matthew's Story

A couple consulted us because they wanted to have a third baby. They had one son aged five. A second little boy was born three years later, with Downs' syndrome. He died when he was three days old. They came for preconceptual counselling but were concerned because they had been given no information about the risks of Downs' syndrome and what they could do to prevent another Downs' baby. We gave them the information on screening which we have included in this chapter. We also estimated the risk of a second Downs' baby. Based on age alone, Jane's risk of carrying a Downs' baby was 1 in 718; however, this risk was doubled (to 1 in 359) because she had already had one Downs' baby. We explained that she would certainly be offered amniocentesis in her next pregnancy, what the risks of the procedure were and discussed some alternative courses of action.

A year later they rang to say that Jane was now pregnant and that they had decided that they would not have amniocentesis. We arranged for a scan for Jane at a specialist centre with expertise in detecting Downs' syndrome: the Harris Birthright Centre at Kings College Hospital in London. To their great relief, the scan was normal and a normal healthy boy, Adam, was born in April that year. The Harris Birthright Centre staff are good at giving advice to women in pregnancy who are unsure about scanning and will accept referrals from anywhere in the country. A letter of introduction from the mother's doctor is preferred.

Two Decisions about Tests

Elaine was happy in her second pregnancy at the age of 30 until she received a letter from the hospital telling her that she had a 'positive' result from her Downs' screening test. This result gave her a risk estimate of one in 130 that the baby had Downs' syndrome, based on a two-marker test. She was offered amniocentesis but was not prepared to accept the risk of inducing miscarriage. As for Jane, we arranged detailed scanning for Elaine which provided her with reassurance. The risk estimate of 129 to one that the baby was normal, combined with the scan which detected no markers of Downs' syndrome, was enough for her and her husband. They realised that these tests did not give them an absolute guarantee but were happier to accept this than to undergo the risks of amniocentesis. In the event the baby, Hannah, was normal.

Decision Chart for Screening

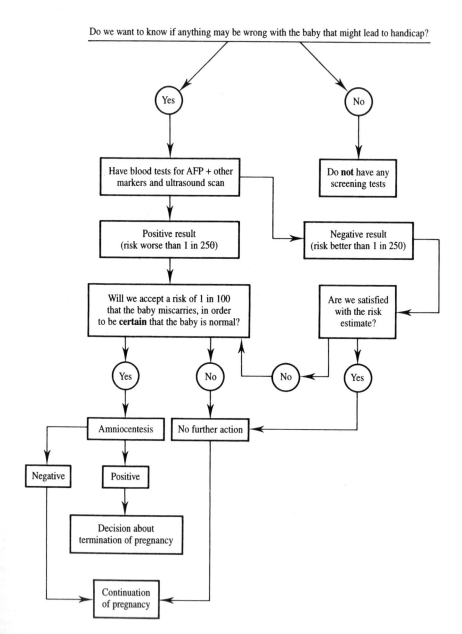

Margaret, at 39, realised that she had an increased risk of a Downs' baby by virtue of her age alone. She was very definite that she could not under any circumstances cope with a Downs' baby. She decided to have amniocentesis whatever the result of her screening. This was done and there were no adverse consequences. The result was a normal karyotype, which means the chromosomes were normal. The baby did not have Downs'. She gave birth to a healthy baby after a normal pregnancy.

A Life Saved by Screening

Vanessa went for a routine scan at 16 weeks in her second pregnancy. The sonographer noticed that the baby had a very rare condition known as gasroschesis. The baby's abdominal wall had not developed properly and the stomach and bowel were outside the baby's body. Vanessa had had her first baby very quickly and safely at home, and was planning another home birth. When the problem was explained to her, she agreed that she would need specialist care for the birth. Her baby was born at full term in hospital and immediately transferred to a regional specialist surgical unit where an operation to repair the defect was performed. Vanessa and her baby are now both perfectly well and healthy. Had the baby been born at home or in hospital without the arrangements being in place for the operation, his chances of survival would have been much reduced.

It must be emphasised that this is a **very** rare condition.

THE MIDDLE THREE MONTHS

....

The time from about 20 to 30 weeks of a pregnancy is relatively quiet as far as the professionals are concerned. All the baby seems to be doing is growing. We are sure, however, that mothers do not feel this way. They become increasingly aware of the baby by feeling movements and noticing the increase in size, along with the discomfort that this may bring. There is also the excitement of the birth getting nearer and the awareness of the reality of the baby. It is a time when mothers ought to take whatever opportunities they have to take care of themselves. Many working mothers will stop work at 26 weeks (though this is not always necessary). Mothers who already have children at home need to try to find some time for themselves.

Feeling the baby move

It is normal to feel the baby move from about 18 to 20 weeks onward. First-time mothers tend to notice this later than those with experience. If you are uncertain about feeling movements at this stage, consult your midwife or doctor. The most probable explanation is that you just don't recognise the movements for what they are and there is nothing to worry about at all, but it's better to get reassurance along these lines and the professionals certainly won't mind giving it. More importantly, if you have already felt movements and find that now you cannot feel them, seek advice as soon as is reasonably practical.

As the movements become stronger it becomes possible for fathers to feel them too by putting a hand on the tummy, and they often feel even more excited than the mothers!

We have noticed an increasing tendency for all sorts of people – friends, relatives and even strangers – to want to touch pregnant mothers' tummies. We don't really understand this but some of our mothers have told us that they find it distressing. Our advice is: this baby is a special intimate gift for its parents. If you don't want other people touching you, stand up for yourself and politely ask them not to do it! 'Please don't do that' might be the appropriate thing to say. People ought to respect the vulnerability and privacy of a mother in pregnancy.

Back Care

About half of all pregnant women experience problems with their backs during pregnancy. This is a huge number of patients, yet midwives and doctors seem unable to help these women. Indeed there has been a tendency to ignore back problems – 'We can't do anything about it, you're pregnant.' About one third of women who have back problems for the first time in pregnancy go on to have a chronic back problem, so we think that it should be taken seriously. Research into ways of preventing and treating back trouble in pregnancy is urgently needed. The middle period of pregnancy is a time when these problems begin to become more apparent and also a time when some action can be taken. Exercises for back care are described in detail in Chapter Six.

The causes of back problems in pregnancy

Hormones: the hormone *progesterone* increases to very high levels in the blood from the moment the baby implants in the uterus. Progesterone causes softening of ligaments (the fibrous tissues that link bones and muscles). This has a useful purpose because it makes the pelvis more flexible in readiness for labour, but the disadvantage for women is that it is much easier to cause a sprain by stretching, bending or lifting during pregnancy.

Posture: as the baby grows, the extra weight tends to throw the centre of gravity of the body forward and causes an increasing forward curve in the lumbar spine (the bottom part of the back). The pelvis then tends to rotate forward to compensate for this, so that the mechanics of the spine and pelvis change. Muscles and ligaments then work in an unfamiliar way and again are more readily damaged by bending, lifting and stretching.

Abdominal stretching: as the uterus grows in size, the abdominal muscles tend to stretch over it. These muscles usually help to maintain the balance of the body and the normal posture and load-bearing position of the spine by acting on the pelvis. As pregnancy progresses, this function is disturbed.

How to take care of your back in pregnancy

Understanding the causes of back pain can lead to action to prevent or treat the problem.

Lax ligaments can't be changed but awareness may result in prevention of damage. Expectant mothers ought to be extra careful about stretching, lifting and bending. Of course it's easy to say and write this, but when you are a mother with small children who want to be picked up, it can be very difficult to put into practice. A job involving lifting may not be possible to change for financial reasons. We all know the correct way to lift, but most of us, without thinking, tend to bend from the waist to pick things up, especially our children. We should bend our knees and lift keeping the back straight. Picking a child out of a cot in the middle of the night is probably the most disastrous movement for the back. Most parents have experienced hearing the cry, groping their way into the room, bending over the cot *without dropping the side*, and lifting out the child, only to feel pain or stiffness in the morning. It doesn't take more than a few seconds to lower the cot side and hopefully do a little to prevent back strain.

Posture With a very little effort it is possible to improve posture during pregnancy and help to prevent back strain. The effort is really a mental rather than a physical one. Remembering to correct posture is the key, and this can be done at all sorts of times during the day – it's not necessary to set aside time for exercises, although this may help too. The following diagram and checklist is reproduced by kind permission of Ronnie Cruwys, an Active Birth Teacher. Many of our mothers have found it helpful.

Posture Checklist

Try and carry out a posture check whenever you are standing ie. answering the telephone, washing up or brushing teeth.

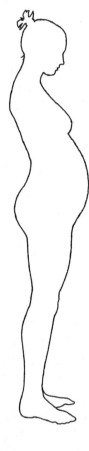

–   Head   +

–	+
If neck sags, chin pokes forward and body slumps.	Straighten neck, tuck in chin so body lines up.

Shoulders/Chest

Slouching cramps ribcage and makes breathing difficult. Arms are turned in.	Lift up through ribcage and pull back shoulder girdle. Roll arms out.

Abdomen/Buttocks

Slack muscles, hollow back, pelvis tilts forward. (Strains back).	Contract abdomen to flatten back. Tuck buttocks under and tilt pelvis back.

Knees

Pressed back, strains joints, pushes pelvis forward.	Bend to ease body weight over feet.

Feet

Weight on inner borders strains arches.	Distribute body weight through centre of each foot.

Strengthening the abdominal muscles

This is a good idea in preparation for labour as well as a preventive measure for back problems. Some simple exercises can help to maintain tone in the abdominal muscles.

Sit comfortably with your feet flat on the floor and back straight. Try to pull in your tummy so that the waistband of your skirt or trousers feels loose. Hold this for a count of two, then relax. Repeat this exercise as often as you can and try to increase the time you hold it. Try to breathe normally while doing this exercise.

Another good exercise is the pelvic tilt, described in Chapter Two.

Physiotherapy and Osteopathy

Physiotherapists and osteopaths have useful roles in the care of pregnant women. Physiotherapy is usually available free on the NHS, but osteopathy is usually not provided by the NHS. Both specialities can be of help in preventing and relieving back pain. Physiotherapy can also be of help in preventing and relieving the distressing condition of stress incontinence which may be a problem during and after pregnancy. Physiotherapists provide advice on care of the perineum. Access to the NHS physiotherapist for mothers is via the GP or midwife. Private physiotherapists may be approached directly, as may osteopaths, but many GPs and midwives now have contacts with local practitioners and would be able to advise mothers on who to consult.

Exercise

Remembering the need for back care in pregnancy, most forms of exercise are good for mothers. Regular exercise has beneficial effects on general health. Firstly, it obviously improves general fitness. Muscles and joints that are used regularly and without excessive or unnatural strain, remain healthy for longer. Secondly, it is of proven benefit to the heart. Regular exercise which increases the heart rate by about ten beats per minute over the norm will help to prevent heart disease. Thirdly, exercise has been proven to benefit the mind and emotions by preventing depression. There's a good common sense reason for this – doing something which releases tension burns up energy and, most importantly, it is enjoyable, and helps us all to feel better about ourselves and our body image. In pregnancy, this can be very important because such great changes are occurring in the mother's body, emotions and social circumstances. First-time mothers especially, when they stop work and, at the same time, find that they are changing shape, may feel low self-esteem. The baby is not here yet, there is nothing to do except watch themselves change, they may feel unattractive and have no sense of purpose. This is the time when regular exercise can have a very beneficial effect both physically and emotionally. If it can be done with a friend or in a group, then there are other benefits too.

What is safe in pregnancy?

We are frequently asked, 'Is it safe to do this?' or to 'keep doing that?' Generally speaking, if a mother has been doing some form of exercise before she became pregnant, then it is safe to continue during the pregnancy. We might discourage more violent or dangerous forms of exercise, especially in late pregnancy, such as hang gliding or martial arts, but with appropriate precautions it may be possible to continue almost any sport if a mother was already used to doing it on a regular basis before. New forms of exercise or sport, however, require more care. This is true for anyone taking up a new sport or exercise. We should take it slowly at first, gradually building up the amount and intensity of the exercise as we become fitter.

Exercise in Water

There has been a great deal of interest in water as a 'treatment' during pregnancy and childbirth in the last ten years. We will discuss water for labour and birth later.

EXERCISE IN WATER

Evidence During the antenatal period, exercise in water has been shown to have several benefits for mothers and their babies.

This exercise can be swimming, but any form of exercise performed in water will have the same beneficial effects. There are now aquanatal classes available at swimming baths in most towns, with a midwife in attendance to advise on exercise for mothers. The benefits are the same as those of 'dry land' exercise but with the additional benefits of greater relaxation – most people feel relaxed in the bath, and just floating and relaxing can make us feel better.

Exercise in water also relieves some of the annoying symptoms of middle and late pregnancy, especially swelling of the hands and feet, and muscle cramps. It has an effect on blood pressure both by the relaxation produced in water and by the induction of diuresis (the kidneys put out more urine which causes a reduction in blood pressure).

Your midwife should be able to tell you where and when aquanatal classes take place. These have the added advantage of being *only* for pregnant mothers. Contact with and support from other mothers can be very helpful from the beginning of pregnancy but especially as it progresses through the middle period. If it's not possible to go to aquanatal classes, then swimming or exercising in an ordinary swimming bath is the next best thing.

Relaxation

Techniques of relaxation training in preparation for birth have been used for many years in antenatal classes. The idea is to practise relaxation methods that can be used during the birth. Relaxation produces pain relief for reasons that will be discussed later. There are many methods of relaxation and no one method is better than any other. The best method is probably the one that best suits the individual mother – what's right for you. It's good for everyone to relax, just as it's good for everyone to exercise, especially in our present stressful life. Five minutes to unwind, out of a busy day of work or child care, can be a wonderful tonic. We'll describe a simple method here, which everyone could try; however, relaxation is a skill which has to be learnt and like all skills, is best learnt from a teacher and, even better still, in a group. Midwives often run relaxation groups in antenatal clinics as part of parentcraft or antenatal classes.

A Simple Relaxation Method for Mothers – Step by Step

1. Find a comfortable chair with a high back so that you can rest your head, or lie down on a bed or the floor.
2. Close your eyes.
3. Stretch out your feet, and lift your legs from the ground a little, just enough to feel the tension in the muscles. Hold the position for a moment, and then lower your legs down to rest.

4. Repeat step 3, feeling the tension, and then relaxing the muscles.
5. Stretch out your arms, stretching all the way to your finger tips, hold the position for a moment, and then rest them down again.
6. Repeat step 5, feeling the tension in your arms, and then relaxing.
7. Clench your teeth tightly and shut your eyes really tight, feel the tension in your face and then relax those muscles.
8. Repeat step 7. By now all your muscles should be relaxed – it is feeling the difference between tension and relaxation that produces the relaxation effect.
9. Concentrate on your breathing, taking slow, gentle breaths, not too deep, relaxing each time you breathe out.
10. Just stay relaxed like this for **five minutes**. Remember, this is time for **you**. Practising like this for five minutes every day really can make a difference.

This method can be combined with meditation if you wish. You might like to focus your thoughts on the baby while you relax. Begin to picture your baby and to feel love for him or her.

If you are a religious person, this method of meditation can become part of your prayers or devotions in any faith. Hold a verse of scripture in your mind as you relax, and feel closer to God. Hold your baby up to him in your prayers.

Relaxation in Water

Almost everyone has had the experience of coming home from work, or finally getting the last child into bed, and thinking 'What I really need is a good long bath!' We rush up to the bathroom, turn on the taps and then at last lie back in the bath and let out a deep sigh. This is a very relaxing everyday experience which can be harnessed for relaxation during pregnancy and in labour (more of which in Chapter Seven).

In preparing for birth, relaxing in water in your own bathroom, which is private and quiet, can be very beneficial. This has some of the physiological benefits of exercise in water – reducing blood pressure and swelling legs – but the emotional and psychological benefits are probably more important. If the bath can be sufficiently full to allow a little floating, this can be very good for relaxation. Floating can be combined with exercise in water in the swimming pool. Just lying on top of the water and allowing the water to massage the skin while breathing slowly and gently can be a very calming experience. This kind of experience is useful in preparation for labour. Like other forms of relaxation it is a skill which is learned by practice. Relaxation can therefore be used in labour even if this does not take place in water. If you are going to use a birthing pool and are able to try it out during the middle part of pregnancy, this too will be a good preparation and help with relaxation when the time comes. The birthing pool contains much more water than the average bath, so floating and relaxing is much easier and freer.

Visualisation is another powerful tool to combine with relaxation, either in water or on land. In the bath, perhaps a picture of the sea and gentle waves may be a calming influence. Everyone has their own particular images which create calm. Maybe the bath is a good place to experiment and find your own. It may also be a good place to visualise the baby who is also floating in water, breathing gently and hearing the sounds of its mother's heartbeat.

Aromatherapy *essential oils* can be used in the bath, but care should be taken about the amount used – it should be only a drop in a bath. Strong oils such as rosemary, thyme, basil, tea tree and myrrh should be avoided in pregnancy according to the aromatherapists. If in doubt, mothers should consult a trained aromatherapist. Oils that certainly can be used safely and which will increase the relaxing effect of a bath are lavender and rose – these are also good for babies and can be used in the birthing pool in labour. Camomile is good for babies too. Jasmine can be used in labour. Other oils that can be used safely in pregnancy are rose geranium, ylang ylang, bergamot, lemon grass, lemon, mandarin, tangerine and neroli, which is said to help prevent stretch marks.

Hypnotherapy

A deeper state of relaxation can be produced by hypnosis, which like the method described above, is a *skill to be learned*. Stage hypnotists use the trick as a form of entertainment, but when used as a tool in health care, hypnosis can be very useful. In pregnancy it can be another aid to relaxation and preparation for birth, and in labour it is possible for mothers to use the skills they have acquired through hypnotherapy training, to produce pain relief for themselves. It must be emphasised that **hypnotherapy is an acquired skill**, like riding a bicycle. If practised regularly it can be turned on quickly and used for instant relaxation or for pain relief. Many midwives and doctors practise hypnotherapy. They see themselves as teachers, helping women to help themselves.

Pain relief in labour can be achieved in two ways through hypnotherapy: deep relaxation, which in itself brings pain relief; and specific methods of suggestion directed at relieving pain – for example, we often suggest a picture to mothers of themselves sitting in a comfortable sun lounger in the garden, with a bucket of ice beside it. A hand placed in the bucket feels cold and this feeling of coldness produces numbness and insensitivity to pain. Placing the 'cold' hand on the part of the body where pain is felt can result in pain relief. Everyone has their own individual best picture which they associate with relaxation or pain relief. For some, a warm feeling is better than cold. The hypnotherapist should find these things out before starting therapy. If you are interested in hypnotherapy for pregnancy or birth, ask your doctor or midwife. If they can't help you themselves, they may well 'know a man (or woman) who can'.

Reflexology

This is a form of therapy in which massage is applied to the feet. The parts of the body are represented by reflex areas in the feet and massage applied to these areas is intended to have a beneficial effect on the corresponding parts. There is some relationship of this philosophy to acupuncture and acupressure. Reflexologists claim to be able to help with some difficult 'minor' problems of pregnancy such as morning sickness, constipation, heartburn and kidney infection. The part of the foot relating to the uterus in reflexology is the 'medial border' or the inside edge of the foot. This is also close to the acupuncture meridian relating to the pelvis and perineum. Midwives and doctors may know local practitioners of reflexology. The British Reflexology Association publishes a register of its members. (See **Addresses**.)

The Growth and Development of the Baby during the Middle Months

This is a period when little apparently seems to be happening. The baby enters a period of growth after the rapid development of the first three months. At 14 weeks, the baby is about three and a half inches long. The face is nearly fully developed and looks like a baby's face. Sometimes it is possible to see the face on an ultrasound scan. By 17 weeks, scans can show that the baby is making breathing movements with its chest. It is actually 'breathing' the amniotic fluid and moves about a pint of fluid in and out of its chest every day. It secretes urine from the kidneys so there is a continuous circulation of amniotic fluid in this way. By 20 weeks, the baby is about ten inches long and is fully formed and developed. The baby is now wriggling and kicking quite a lot, and may start to suck his or her thumb.

Changing Shape

If the baby has not been noticeable until 16 to 18 weeks, it certainly will become more obvious during the middle months. Some mothers regard this as a positive experience, thriving on the 'blooming' pregnant appearance. Many, however, feel badly about themselves because of the increase in size and weight. Perhaps our society's value of the slim figure contributes to these negative feelings. It's important to try to feel good about oneself in pregnancy, to 'maintain a positive self-image'. We suggest three strategies for doing this.

Firstly, when you start to have negative thoughts about size and shape, tell yourself that this is a temporary change and that after the baby is born, you will regain your usual figure. The temporary change is a good one, because the result will be the baby.

Secondly, think that your negative view of yourself is a distortion of reality, and as such, try to put it out of your mind. It may be easier to do this if you remember that this state is temporary.

Thirdly, remember that we don't see ourselves as others see us. Our view of ourself may be, for example, of someone who is fat and misshapen, but others may see us very differently. We tend to weigh our own opinions of how we look more highly than those of others. Try to build up evidence from what other people, valued by you, think about how you look in pregnancy. Usually they will say, honestly, that you look good. Try to give this more importance than your own negative view.

Weight Gain

In a normal pregnancy a mother can expect to gain between 9.6 and 19.2 kilos, or 20 to 40 pounds. There is not much weight gain to start with, but as the baby grows, so the weight gain increases. 39% of the increase is the baby, 22% is from the increase in the volume of the mother's blood, 11% each from the uterus and the amniotic fluid, 9% from the placenta and 8% from the increase in breast tissue. There is no 'normal' pattern of weight gain and we do not believe that weighing mothers frequently is helpful. An awareness of the normality of gaining weight and sticking to a good diet (see Chapters One and Two) is all that is necessary.

Clothes

Because the change in shape is now becoming obvious, mothers may become concerned about their clothes at this stage in the pregnancy. If you're fortunate enough to be able to afford a new wardrobe every six months, then the latest in maternity wear can be yours. Special maternity clothes won't be used for long though – at most for four months, and even if you are already planning another pregnancy, the time of year may be different for the next one. Many mothers have told us that they can get by without maternity wear with some very simple loose-fitting clothes such as large T-shirts with leggings, or loose-fitting dresses. One important point is that the breasts tend to enlarge quite markedly from early pregnancy. A well-fitting bra is important to keep comfortable. These are available from the major chain stores dealing with maternity wear and equipment, such as Mothercare and Boots. There is usually information on the packet explaining how to estimate the likely size you will need, taking account of your size before pregnancy. These bras are available for pregnancy or for nursing, or there is an all-in-one type that can be used for both. If in doubt, find a friend with previous, recent experience and discuss it with her.

Problems in the Middle Months

The period between 10 to 30 weeks tends to be a 'quiet' one in pregnancy, when little seems to be happening except for growth, but mothers may experience some symptoms of pregnancy which can be a real nuisance during this time. Mothers shouldn't be afraid to bring these apparently 'trivial' complaints to the attention of their midwives or doctors. They ought to be taken seriously as they can cause a lot of misery.

Indigestion
This often becomes more apparent because of hormonal changes and the growth of the uterus, disorting the anatomy of the stomach. Many women

describe this as 'heartburn' – a burning sensation in the middle of the chest, which is triggered or made worse by eating or bending or lying down. This can cause loss of sleep and be very distressing.

Avoiding spicy foods and those postures which bring on the symptom are the obvious first remedies. If this is not enough, and for most women it probably isn't, antacid mixtures should be tried. The cheapest is 'Milk of Magnesia', which is available from pharmacists or can be prescribed by doctors as Magnesium Trisilicate. Some antacids act by forming a 'raft' on the surface of the stomach, thus protecting the oesophagus (gullet) from acid refluxing from the stomach. The two most commonly used are Gaviscon and Gastrocote – also available from chemists or on prescription. Some women, however, don't respond to these alkalis which ought to neutralise the stomach acid, and for them, weak *acids* seem to work better. There is research **evidence** that this is an effective treatment, although it seems illogical that acid could make an acid problem better. The hydrochloric acid in the stomach is so strong that a weaker acid may actually reduce its effect. Lemon juice is such a weak acid. If you don't get any relief from the antacids, try some. Homoeopathic causticum can also relieve heartburn, especially when *burning* is the predominant symptom.

Gentle massage to the spinal muscles below and between the shoulder blades can help relieve heartburn. This can be done by a friend or partner and is also very relaxing. A trick for self-help is to roll a hand towel from both ends to form two sausages that can rest lengthways on either side of the spine, just below the shoulder blades. Lean back against a firm chair to apply a steady pressure to the muscles in the spine. Relaxing these muscles influences the nerves coming from this part of the spine which influence digestion.

Constipation

This can cause considerable discomfort in pregnancy but has a more serious consequence if left untreated, because for those subject to *piles*, pregnancy and constipation together can result in worsening this painful condition.

Constipation can be prevented by diet, adequate fluid intake and regular exercise. The foods that help to prevent constipation are those containing *fibre*. These include fresh fruit and vegetables, wholemeal bread and pasta and pulses. Many people feel that it is better to take a wholefood diet containing plenty of these foods, than to supplement fibre in the diet by adding bran.

If simple measures don't work, then it may be necessary to take laxatives. Preferably these should be natural bulking agents such as lactulose or Fybogel. Laxatives, such as senna, which stimulate the bowel can result in stomach cramps and if used frequently, they may cause fluid loss which weakens the mother. Effects on the baby are unknown, but these stimulant laxatives are known to cross the placenta and go into the baby's bloodstream, so they are best avoided. Early advice from midwife or doctor may avoid problems associated with constipation if the dietary measures above are not sufficient. A prescription for a natural laxative such as Fybogel or Lactulose, which are not absorbed into the mother's blood and therefore cannot harm either mother or baby, may help.

Massage to the dorsal and lumbar muscles, and gentle abdominal massage can help constipation. A friend or partner would have to do the back massage, but abdominal massage can be done yourself. Put your right hand on your tummy, on the right, just above the hip, and gently massage in a clockwise direction, upwards and round and down towards the left hip. This follows the course of the large intestine.

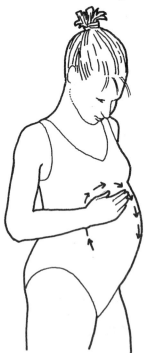

The direction of rub in abdominal massage.

Problems with Sleeping

There are a number of troublesome physical problems which may start to cause loss of sleep for mothers in the middle of pregnancy. There's no need to put up with these, as remedies can usually be found which do not involve the use of drugs.

We've already talked about heartburn or indigestion. Acid production by the stomach is at its greatest during the night, so these problems are often more troublesome then and wake mothers from sleep. The antacid tablets or medicine can be taken last thing at night to prevent these symptoms waking you up. The dose at bedtime should be larger than that taken in the day – three tablets of antacid or 15ml of medicine instead of two tablets or 10ml. Tea, coffee and alcohol stimulate acid production, so these should be avoided at bedtime. Food also stimulates acid production so although there may be immediate relief of symptoms by taking a snack at bedtime, you're likely to pay for it in the middle of the night.

Other problems can be night cramps and fetal movements. Cramp can often be resolved by simple measures such as making sure that you get adequate fluid balance during the day – because of the bladder symptoms which tend to get worse in the later part of pregnancy, mothers may not actually drink enough fluid during the day. Massage can relieve and prevent cramp, and if this fails we have found that a drink of Indian tonic water at bedtime often does the trick. We think it works because tonic contains a small amount of quinine which is used to treat cramps. The amount in a glass of tonic water is insufficient to have any effect on the baby, but our mothers tell us that it works for their cramps. Homoeopathic cinchona can have the same effect and is safe. Other homoeopathic remedies may be effective, but at this stage you would need the help of a homoeopath.

There's not much to be done about fetal movements. In fact, no one would want to stop them because they indicate a live healthy baby. The baby unfortunately doesn't seem to know the time and may choose to be awake when the mother wants to sleep. Perhaps knowing that the baby is there and awake and healthy might be a reassuring feeling which would induce sleep. If you're kept awake by movements, maybe you could try thinking this way. If it's anxious thoughts that keep you awake as well as the movements, the best advice is: don't lie in bed feeling and thinking. Get up, walk about, have a cup of tea or whatever drink appeals, then go back to bed when you feel tired again.

We think it is best not to take sleeping tablets of any kind during pregnancy because all pharmaceutical hypnotics cross the placenta and affect the baby. A warm drink last thing at night (but not coffee or chocolate which contain caffeine), a good book or some relaxation exercises or self-hypnosis can be useful ways of getting off to sleep. Homoeopathic coffea may help, taken at bedtime, or consult a homoeopath for your 'constitutional remedy'.

Swelling in Hands and Feet

The technical term is oedema. It can start in the middle months, but is at its worst in the last two months. There is no serious medical significance of swelling hands and feet in pregnancy. It is another unfortunate but normal phenomenon. It can be prevented to some extent by exercise in water. Walking is good, but standing still for more than a few minutes at a time tends to make things much worse. Support tights or stockings provide relief, as does simple immersion in a bath of warm water – although the effect may not last very long. Herbal teas, in particular those made from bearberry, buchu and dandelion, have helped some of our mothers with this problem.

Massaging the feet is very relaxing (see *Reflexology*) and calf-stretching exercises (see Chapter Two) can help reduce the fluid in the feet and legs by encouraging flow back to the body.

Tightness in the pectoral muscles in the chest can contribute to hand swelling. A simple exercise to stretch the pectorals is to 'walk' your fingers up a wall as far as you can reach, hold for ten seconds and gradually bring your arms down. Repeat this about ten times or until you feel less of a stretch in the chest. **This should not hurt. If it does, stop**.

Itching

This can be a real nuisance and is quite a common occurrence. The itching can be on any part of the body, but it seems more common on the abdomen. Sometimes it affects the whole body. There may be a rash, but often there is nothing to see on the skin. Wearing loose clothes made of natural fibres may help to prevent or alleviate the problem. Calamine lotion is the first thing to try for relief. Antihistamine tablets should only be used if the problem is really driving you crazy, and it would be best to get these on prescription from your doctor. Homoeopathic remedies can help too but it would be best to consult a homoeopath or homoeopathic doctor for advice. A very rare but serious condition called cholestasis of pregnancy, which affects the liver, may cause severe itching in the last three months of pregnancy.

Twins

The use of ultrasound scanning now means that twins are usually detected in the early part of pregnancy. In the middle months, the uterus will certainly begin to be bigger than for a single pregnancy. As the babies grow, so there will be extra stresses on the mother's body. A mother of twins needs more rest. The same advice about exercise, especially exercise in water, applies just as much to mothers of twins as to mothers of single babies. It is even more important for mothers of twins to do pelvic floor exercises (see Chapter Six) because of the greater strain placed on these muscles by the extra baby. Back care is also more important.

There is a higher risk of high blood pressure, anaemia and of premature labour. It is wise for mothers of twins to be cared for in a consultant unit because of the greater risk of complications during the pregnancy and at the birth. Some obstetricians like to admit mothers of twins to hospital for rest between 30 and 36 weeks. Mothers with children at home may well find this difficult and doctors and midwives should understand this. If there are no complications making a stay in hospital essential, it should be possible to organise rest at home with the help of family and friends, but this should be more than just an hour or two in the day with the feet up.

Hydramnios (or Polyhydramnios)

This means too much fluid around the baby and is a more common complication of twin pregnancies. It can develop very suddenly (acute hydramnios) or can build up slowly. Many cases are mild and need nothing more than a careful professional watching by a consultant. If hydramnios becomes more serious, you may need admission for rest because of the risk of premature labour.

Cervical Incompetence

A relatively unusual cause of miscarriage in the middle months of pregnancy, typically between 18 and 26 weeks, is described by the term cervical incompetence, although the exact mechanism by which this occurs is not known. The idea behind the phrase 'cervical incompetence' is that a miscarriage results from the neck of the womb, or cervix, becoming slack, thus allowing the baby to 'fall out' and deliver early.

The chances of survival of such an early birth are virtually negligible, though babies have been known to survive when born as early as 22 weeks.

CERVICAL INCOMPETENCE

Evidence An operation to strengthen the cervix, by the insertion of a suture or stitch (known as a *Schirodkar suture* or a *McDonald suture*), is effective for some women. Women more likely to benefit from this procedure are those who have had two or more miscarriages at this stage of pregnancy. For other women, the risks of surgery and of actually stimulating early labour by the insertion of the stitch, outweigh any possible benefits and this procedure is therefore **not recommended** for such women.

Lynette had one uncomplicated pregnancy and normal birth and was pregnant again two years later when, at 20 weeks, she went into labour and, of course, miscarried, the baby being too small to survive. After this dreadful experience, Lynette was full of questions which we could not answer satisfactorily. What had caused the miscarriage? Was there anything she could have done to prevent it? Would it happen again? She had some infection after the first pregnancy, did that have anything to do with it? Naturally, in her grief, she tended to blame herself, although she knew this was irrational. After another 18 months, she became pregnant again, and after discussion with a specialist, she had a McDonald suture inserted at 12 weeks. It was removed at 36 weeks and she went into labour two weeks later and gave birth to Lydia, a healthy girl.

CHAPTER SIX

LATE PREGNANCY – THE LAST THREE MONTHS

....

From 30 weeks onwards, the arrival of a new baby seems to get closer, and more real. From what our mothers tell us, there seem to be both positive and negative sides to this growing reality. On the one hand, there's the sense of being 'nearly there'. It's good to start preparing for the birth at the beginning of this phase, remembering that normal labour can start between 37 and 42 weeks. On the other hand, problems associated with the increasing size and weight of the baby begin to occur now.

Preparation for Birth

We think preparation should involve thinking about four 'Ps'. **Place, People, Position** and **Pain Relief**. Most mothers have probably chosen the **place** for their baby's birth by now – at home or in hospital, in a GP or Midwifery unit or in a Consultant unit.

However, **it's not too late to change your mind!** In fact, it's never too late, but there's no doubt that the outcome of birth for both mother and baby is better when there has been planning of the place of birth beforehand. It must be more secure emotionally for a mother to give birth in the place she has already chosen. If you're reading this and you feel unsure about where you'd like to give birth to your baby, why not go back to Chapter Three and work through the decision chart. It might help to clarify your thoughts, to make you more settled as to your choice, or to help you to make a different choice. Your midwives and doctors should not mind your change of heart; after all, **it's your body and your baby**. Having settled on the place, you need to make it as comfortable for you as possible.

Preparing your Home for a Home Birth

Decide first of all which room you will use. This may be governed by many factors, but probably overriding all is: where do you feel most relaxed and comfortable? It need not necessarily be the bedroom, but if you feel most relaxed and comfortable in or near your own bed, then that's the place. If you are going to use a birthing pool, then it's probably better downstairs because of the weight of water needed to fill the pool – about 200 gallons which weigh nearly ten hundredweight. If you live above the ground floor, for example in a flat or maisonette, or if you want to take the pool upstairs, take advice about the strength of the floor joists. If you're sure the joists will take it, and the facilities for filling the pool are close enough, and if upstairs feels best to you, then it's OK.

Privacy is another important consideration. Many mothers feel that they don't want to be disturbed during labour and feel an intense need for privacy, so choose a room where this can be achieved. You may want to consider the room as your environment for birth. What about lighting, smells, things you want around you to make a more relaxed environment? Music can be particularly helpful to produce relaxation so make sure you have access to your favourite tapes, records or CDs. Some mothers, on the other hand, prefer silence, so try to think how this can be best achieved. Think whether you will prefer dim lighting or lots of light. Would some scents be relaxing? Some mothers find aromatherapy oils burnt in a candle lamp helpful. What sort of food and drink would you like to have ready? (Don't forget the midwife and doctor too!) Labour can go on for some time, and can use up a good deal of energy, so it's good to have high energy foods, carbohydrates in particular, ready. Instruct the people who will be with you how to make your favourites if they don't already know. If you are going to give birth in your own home you should have complete control over all this, but when in labour, of course, mothers find that they have to concentrate on what is happening to themselves, so preparation beforehand is wise.

Equipment for Home Birth

Your midwife will bring all the technical equipment needed for a birth (and there's not very much of that). We advise our mothers to have a plastic sheet to protect the bed or wherever else is planned for the birth, some old sheets, and some towels for herself and the baby. A few first baby clothes are a good idea, but not absolutely essential, and a few first-size nappies.

Preparing for Hospital Birth

Hospital is an unfamiliar environment. Unfamiliarity prevents relaxation. To counter this problem, if you have chosen to have a hospital birth, make yourself as familiar with the environment in which you will give birth as possible. Most maternity hospitals arrange tours for mothers and fathers in the evenings. Your midwife should know when these will take place. If you can't go to a tour or open evening, then you should still be able to visit the labour ward by prior arrangement with the staff. Preparation for birth in this way is most important, and mothers tell us that even a brief trip round the hospital in the company of a midwife helps enormously to allay anxieties. It also helps to have met the hospital staff because a familiar face is another relaxing factor in labour. The best familiar face is your own midwife or family doctor who may be able to attend you in labour, but this is not always possible in the hospital units, so try to get to know the people who will be looking after you at the birth.

As you look round the hospital, try to imagine yourself in labour in this place. What will you use to lean on if you need something to support your weight? What cushions could you bring in to help you make this more comfortable? Remember that the longer you can keep mobile and upright during labour, the better. This will help both you and the baby (see Chapter Seven). How will you be able to do this? Where will you be able to walk around?

Sometimes labour will slow down after the move to hospital, and the mother then may need a private place where she can relax and be quiet for a while. Is there such a place that you could go to if this happens? A bathroom may be the answer. Anticipating these situations when visiting the hospital may well help mothers to feel more in control when they are in labour and find themselves in hospital.

Make the Place Your Own

Hospitals are now very aware of the need for a relaxed environment for birth and try to make even the most technological of units feel as homely as possible by means of decoration and allowing music and belongings to be brought in. Plan to bring in your own CD or cassette player with music if this helps you, a few familiar and favourite soft furnishings such as rugs or cushions, your favourite pictures or photographs if they are reasonably portable, and your candles or aromatherapy lamps if these help. Check with the hospital what is 'OK' if you've any doubts. Most will be highly accommodating. Try to make the place as much your own space as is possible.

Checklist of Things to Take With You to Hospital

Your local hospital probably has its own list which should be provided in an information pack given to you when you first meet your midwife, or in the antenatal clinic. Hospitals vary in what they provide for mothers, so it's best to check their own list. Here are some of the basics you may need in addition to the 'homemaking' things discussed in the last section:

For Yourself
- Two or three night-dresses, preferably front-opening
- Dressing gown and slippers
- Two bras
- One bath towel, one hand towel
- Shower cap
- Two flannels
- Soap
- Toothbrush and toothpaste
- Brush, comb and shampoo
- Make-up
- Paper tissues
- Sanitary pads and belt. Tampons can't be used after the birth because they may be painful or cause infection
- Books or a Walkman or other entertainment items
- Notelets
- Coins for the telephone or a phonecard

For the Baby
- Towel
- Nappies
- Baby clothes

People

Who would you like with you during the labour and at the birth? Think about this in your preparation. Research evidence shows that the most important influence on the outcome of labour for both mother and baby is the presence of a trusted, familiar person throughout. This factor far outweighs any medical or midwifery influences. The support person does not even have to be experienced in midwifery or medicine to have this beneficial influence. It is natural to assume that your husband or partner will be present at the birth. He may be the trusted, familiar support person, or it may be someone else, a friend, sister or mother.

The involvement of men in birth has been very much a late twentieth-century, western development. While this is not to be decried, it must be recognised that many cultures in the past and at present, in other parts of the world, exclude men from birth. Traditionally in Britain, men paced the floor outside during the birth. Our experience is that few want to do this and that few women wish their men away from the birth of their children, but we feel that social pressure should not result in either women or men feeling uncomfortable because the men are *expected* to take part. The support of women for women in labour should not be underestimated. It may be that you would prefer to have two supporters with you in labour, your husband or partner and a friend or other close relative. It may be that you want to have one of your children present. Hospitals have a natural resistance to non-professionals, especially children, being around, but there has been much more flexibility in recent years and so it should be possible to negotiate what you want.

Which professionals would you like to be present? Which midwife, which doctor, if they are involved? The ideal is for your Community Midwife, who has looked after you throughout the pregnancy, and who you know and trust, to be your main birth attendant. This may not always be possible, but if it is, do you feel most comfortable with this midwife? If you happen to meet a midwife with whom you can't get on, then ask for a change. This is your right. The Health Authority or Hospital Trust **must** provide you with another midwife if you ask them. If your doctor is involved with birth and can be at the birth, do you want him or her? If not, say not! If you have a complicated pregnancy and require consultant care, do you feel comfortable about the doctors who will look after you? If not, ask your family doctor to arrange for a different consultant.

All these choices are open to mothers and always have been, but only since the publication of 'Changing Childbirth' (the 1994 Government report on Maternity Services) have they been explicitly expressed as Health Service policy. This should make it even easier now for mothers to obtain the care they feel most comfortable with.

Position

It is simple common sense that an upright position must be best for birth since gravity will help the contractions of the uterus. Conversely, lying on one's back on the bed in the 'traditional' position cannot allow gravity to help.

POSITION

Evidence Research has established that our common sense is right and that any position other than lying on the back on a bed gives better results and easier, quicker labour.

All hospitals, doctors and midwives know this but in all branches of health care it is difficult to change established practice; we know that mothers are still encouraged to give birth lying on beds in a disadvantageous position. Practising for a good position before labour starts will not only help you to prepare for birth but also to overcome any objections from your birth attendants.

Any position which is comfortable, other than lying on your back, is good

Sitting up on the bed, although better than lying on the back, still has disadvantages. The reasons for this are related to your anatomy. Lying down, the baby has actually to travel upwards through the birth canal, therefore gravity is working against the contractions of the uterus. In this position, the pelvis is restricted and cannot open to its widest points to allow the delivery of the baby's head. The bones at the back of the pelvis, the sacrum and coccyx, are restricted and cannot move to allow the head to pass. Sitting up in bed overcomes gravity but there is still the problem of restriction of the sacrum and coccyx. The best natural positions for labour are a 'supported squat', kneeling on all fours, or lying on the side.

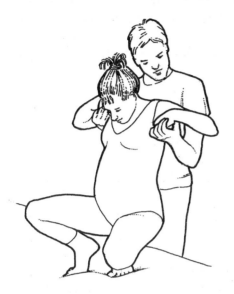

Partner stands behind the bed while the mother squats.

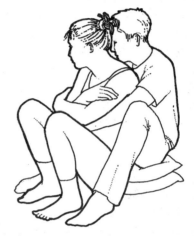

The mother squats between her partner's knees. He sits on the bean-bag behind her.

Practising squatting

If you are going to use the supported squat in labour, it is a good plan to practise the position a few times beforehand. Some exercises will help to prepare for using this position and also help to open the pelvis to its widest point and help the flexibility of the pelvic floor and ligaments.

If you have piles (see later in this chapter) or varicose veins in the vulva, or have had a cervical stitch, it would be best to do these exercises with the support of a stool, or even better, and for greater comfort, a bucket for support. Since we learnt from one mother how she had used a bucket, placed right way up, to sit on for comfort in the later part of pregnancy and during labour, many of our mothers have tried it with success!

- ◆ Practise squatting with the help of a partner, or with something firm to support your weight, such as a heavy table or a window ledge.

- ◆ Stand with feet apart and firmly planted on the ground.
- ◆ Breathe in deeply.
- ◆ As you breathe out, bend your knees and allow your pelvis to drop between your knees, holding on to your partner, or other support.
- ◆ Spread your knees as wide as possible.
- ◆ With each outbreath, allow your shoulders and the muscles in your back to relax.
- ◆ Let your bottom almost touch your heels.
- ◆ Hold the position for a few breaths, then slowly come back to standing.

Pain Relief

This 'P' has been left till last because it depends to a very large extent on the first two. The first line of pain relief is to feel relaxed and comfortable in the place you want to be in, in the company of people you feel you trust. The effect of these factors is surprisingly strong. We know this instinctively from childhood because when a child falls and hurts itself the first thing he or she wants is to be with Mummy or Daddy. The next demand is usually, 'I want to go home.' Getting place and people right will help with the pain.

Relaxation is the next line of pain relief. It is not merely that feeling relaxed helps us to cope better with pain, or acts as a distraction from the pain, although both these are true. Relaxation helps to relieve pain by allowing the body to release its own natural pain relievers. These are known as *endorphins*. They are chemicals found in the human brain which are similar to one of the strongest pain killers we know – morphine. Anxiety and tension inhibits release of these natural pain relievers; relaxation encourages their release.

Preparing for Relaxation in Labour

Simple measures encourage relaxation in labour. Firstly, we're back to place and people again. It's a common experience that we feel more relaxed in familiar surroundings that are comfortable to us. It is very individual. Some people, for example, feel more relaxed amid chaos and untidiness whereas others cannot feel relaxed until the room they are in has been tidied up. We want to emphasise that in preparing for labour at home or in hospital, mothers should try to make the place where they will be in labour as comfortable and personal to them as possible. They should have people with them who they can feel relaxed with, and trust, and it follows that if there are people who want to be present at the birth who have the opposite effect, they should be told to stay away (even if these are professionals!).

We know from our mothers, that when they are in labour, it is very difficult to say that a certain person is making them feel anxious, and they'd rather that person was outside the room. Sometimes student midwives or doctors will want to be present at a birth. They need to gain experience but the mother's feelings should take precedence over this. Think this through beforehand because we know that mothers in labour are very vulnerable and will usually agree to anything. If you don't feel you want this sort of intrusion, say so, and get it written in case notes too.

Practising relaxation techniques during pregnancy will help during labour. It's a skill that needs to be learnt and practised so that it can used when required. Hypnotherapy is also a skill which requires practice.

Massage

Touching and rubbing the spot that hurts is a natural human reaction to pain, both for ourselves and for others. Partners can prepare for labour by practising massage, especially of the lower back, and this can be very useful indeed; remember, however, that some mothers prefer to curl up in a ball and not to be touched by anyone, so if you're a partner reading this, prepare for both eventualities.

Get your partner to practise massage by placing a hand each side of the spine, just below the ribs. The pain of early labour tends to be in this area. It moves down towards the pelvis as labour progresses. Can he feel any areas that are tenser than the others? If not, take a deep breath in and out. This may make muscle tension more apparent. If there still aren't any 'hot spots', bend forward a little. One side may move more than the other. The less mobile side is the tense side. If he still can't feel any tension, either you've got a very good back, or you need the help of an osteopath. Get him to work at the tense areas, exerting quite a bit of pressure, but not enough to make it uncomfortable. The massaging movement can be up and down on the skin or a circular movement, whatever feels better. It is usually easier and more effective to apply steady pressure with the thumb to the tender or tight areas. Pressure should be applied gradually and released gradually (easy on and easy off). A rapid on/off pressure is more likely to keep the muscle tight rather than to relax it.

Doing this for long periods in labour can be quite tiring for the partner's hands, so practise beforehand will help. It may help to use a little oil: olive oil, baby oil or aromatherapy oil. Massage can be relaxing and pleasing as well as relieving pain. It is not a 'confidence trick'. There are good theoretical reasons why massage helps relieve pain. It probably works like TENS (see below) in releasing endorphins and using the 'pain gate' theory. There is also a relationship with acupuncture and acupressure – working in the meridians of the body and interfering in a positive way with the energy flow in the body. Relieving muscle tension in itself relieves pain.

Preparation for more specific methods of pain relief

Perhaps mothers reading this will be a little surprised to find that we've talked a lot already about pain relief but have not yet mentioned drugs or other medical methods. Drugs can be useful, but are the last line of defence. In preparation for labour, our mothers find it helpful to talk about the various drugs that are used and to prepare themselves to use them. We'll discuss these in the chapter on labour itself.

Tens

There is another medical method of pain relief which does not need drugs and that is TENS or transcutaneous electrical nerve stimulation. It involves passing a small electrical current through the body near the site of the pain. There are two reasons why this works. Firstly, it is known to release endorphins (see above); secondly, it is thought to stimulate the pain pathways in the body, the nerves that carry pain impulses to the brain by which we recognise that we are in pain. This confuses the brain so that the original pain is no longer perceived. Some mothers have found this method of pain relief to be all they require in labour.

TENS needs planning beforehand if you want to try it in labour. It is given by a small device about the size of a small pocket torch, attached to the body by two or four electrodes. It needs a little practice if it is to be used in labour, because the positioning of the electrodes is important. It has the advantages of portability and absence of side effects. It has no effect on the baby. It cannot, of course, be used in water.

If this seems like a useful idea, discuss it with the midwife or doctor, or with a physiotherapist, and arrange to try out a machine. Some hospitals have machines available for loan, and they can be hired from private companies for relatively small sums.

When you try TENS:

– make sure you are familiar with the controls. Models differ. Most have an 'on/off' switch which is also the intensity (volume) control. Some units have a frequency control too and some a 'boost' button which can be pressed for extra relief when the contraction reaches its peak;
– make sure you have a new battery (most use 9 volt pp3 batteries);
– get whatever tape you need to fix the electrodes in place. Some units are supplied with disposable electrodes which are self-adhesive, and this is the type we prefer, but others need tape to fix electrodes in place. Make sure you are not allergic to the tape you will use.

For use in labour:

– connect the leads to the electrodes;
– apply gel to the electrodes if they are not of the disposable type;
– place the electrodes on your back (someone else will have to do this!);
– the upper electrodes should be level with the tenth thoracic vertebra;
– the lower electrodes should be level with the dimples at the bottom of your back which are over the sacral spine;
– the electrodes should be about three inches apart;
– switch on and turn up the intensity until a *comfortable* sensation can be felt;
– the 'boost' button can be used when the contractions are strong or extra pain relief is needed.

TIP

Only the mother should control the intensity switch. Don't let anyone else touch it!

Don't use TENS:
– if you have a cardiac pacemaker;
– on your abdomen or on any other part of the body except the back as described above;
– in water;
– while driving.

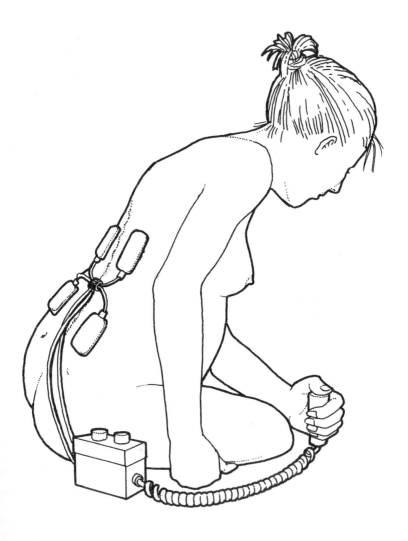

Electrode placement when using a TENS machine.

Safety: The only side effects of TENS are skin burns which may occur with excessive stimulation with small electrodes or poor electrical contact. If the instructions are followed correctly these should never occur.

Judy had a GP unit birth for her second pregnancy. Sadly, the baby, Adam, had a congenital heart problem and died when only eight days old during an operation to try to correct the heart lesion. Judy asked for a home birth for her next baby and was interested in using TENS. We supplied her with our surgery TENS machine. The time came. She rang to say that her contractions had started. When I arrived at the house in the early evening, Judy was ironing. When she had finished the ironing, we applied the TENS electrodes and she began to use the machine for pain relief. Judy used no other form of pain relief throughout her labour. Most of the time she spent walking around her house, and as the contractions grew stronger she clung to her husband in a dancing position. All the time she was increasing the intensity of the TENS and using the boost button as she needed it. Matthew was born at just after midnight. We asked a paediatrician to visit during the first week because of Adam's problem. Matthew is perfectly healthy.

Pain-relieving drugs

It is a good idea to think about the various pharmaceutical drugs that can be used for pain relief in labour and to ask questions about them. What are the side effects? How often should they be given? What are the effects on the baby? These and other questions that may occur to you may not be easily asked when you are in labour and wanting something to relieve the pain. Similar questions can be asked about epidurals, which in theory can produce a pain-free labour. This will be discussed in detail in the next chapter. If you decide on this method, prepare by being aware of the advantages and disadvantages and feeling secure in your decision.

Back Care in Late Pregnancy

In the last part of pregnancy, the extra weight of the baby, the uterus and the amniotic fluid produces a marked alteration in the shape of the spine and in the centre of gravity of the mother. These changes should be easily accommodated by a healthy spine, but often our lifestyles result in us adopting anatomically disadvantageous positions.

A good example is sitting at a word processor or computer screen as I am doing now. I am conscious of the strain on my back, even though I am sitting and not performing strenuous work. As I move to adopt a more sensible posture, and position myself over the keyboard so that my back is straighter and my hands move more freely over the keys in an attitude more like that of a pianist, I can feel instant relief! Such simple adaptations at home or at work could prevent a large number of the back problems among both men and women that family doctors deal with each day.

If you do have back trouble, and have not taken any action about it yet, **act now**. Caring for a new baby may well involve you in a lot of lifting and bending and adoption of unusual postures. Consult your midwife or doctor, or better still physiotherapist or osteopath. Some simple exercises at this stage can help to prevent back problems later. We'll describe three that can be done easily at home, but for more details, consult the experts.

Back-care Exercises for Late Pregnancy

Care of the back involves giving attention to muscles, bones and ligaments surrounding the back as well as those in the back itself. It is important to maintain good movement in all these structures during this part of pregnancy, as problems can often develop from the alterations in posture brought about by the increasing size of the baby and from asymmetry resulting from this change in size and shape. Keeping your body flexible will help as your posture changes, letting your weight be supported by the muscles and ligaments without straining them.

We describe some exercises below. These can be used both to relieve troublesome symptoms, but also as prevention. If the exercises do not help the symptoms, or if they make them worse, **seek professional help** either from your doctor or midwife, or from a registered osteopath or physiotherapist.

Try to keep the following areas supple and flexible:

The chest and shoulders
Tension in the pectoral muscle can be a cause of 'pins and needles' as well as finger swelling. Follow the stretching exercise in Chapter Two.

The lower part of the rib cage and lower back
These exercises can help to relieve or avoid backache, indigestion, constipation and shortness of breath resulting from the baby growing and restricting the mother's breathing.

1.   Sitting, rest your hands on your lower ribs, fingers pointing forwards, thumbs backwards around the ribs. Breathe in deeply, then right out. Compress the ribs with your hands so that all the air is squeezed out. Breathe in but keep the pressure on with your hands for a count of five, then relax and breathe out. Breathe normally and deeply several times before repeating the exercise.

2.   Standing, with legs slightly apart, slowly bend to the left at the same time breathing in and raising the right arm above your head. Run the left hand down the side of your left leg as you do this, so that you can 'push off' with it to return to the upright position. Breathe out as you return to upright. Repeat with the right side, and then repeat both sides about ten times each.

3.   Standing, lift both arms above your head as you breathe in, stretching towards the ceiling. Breathe out as you lower your arms. Repeat about ten times.

The hips

Free hip movement helps the lower back and pelvis to adjust to changes in weight bearing and posture.

Stand with one foot raised on a chair placed against the wall. As you breathe in deeply, lean forward, stretching the muscles around the hips. As you breathe out, lean backwards and relax, then repeat this, taking the stretch a little further forward each time. Repeat using the other leg. Do the whole sequence about ten times.

The calves

These exercises may help to relieve or avoid calf and foot tension. Keeping these muscles relaxed will help fluid drainage from the legs and reduce the risk of varicose veins.

Stand facing a wall. Put your hands just above your head, palms facing the wall, and on to the wall (in a position as though you were about to be 'frisked' by the police!). With feet firmly rooted to the ground, allow your pelvis to lean in. You should feel your calves stretching, and also your lumbar spine. Repeat this about ten times.

The feet

General massage to the feet can be relaxing as well as beneficial in keeping the muscle and ligaments flexible. It is best done by a partner. Special attention might be paid to the acupressure points that are described in Chapter Five.

Exercise for Preparing for Labour

The supported squat is one of the most advantageous positions for giving birth since gravity is harnessed to help the process and the anatomy of the pelvis is used to advantage. This exercise helps to prepare for this position and to strengthen the abdominal muscles in preparation for labour.

Stand with your back touching a wall. Try to get all of the lower part of your back in contact with the wall by pulling in your tummy muscles. Check this by seeing if you can put your hands behind your back. If you can, try to straighten up some more.

Now bend your knees and slowly slide down the wall into a squatting position, and then straighten the knees and slowly come back to standing. Repeat this about eight times. It should be possible to do this exercise daily without it hurting. **If it hurts, don't do it**.

Pelvic Floor Exercises

A number of women suffer from incontinence of urine after birth. This can be very distressing and embarrassing, and we find that women often don't mention it to their medical attendants because they are so embarrassed. Strengthening the pelvic floor muscles can help to prevent this distressing condition. Some simple exercises can help. They are easy to do and should be practised every day. We think all pregnant mothers should do this.

The Pelvic Floor

This is a very good description of the layers of muscles which support all the organs in the pelvis – it is literally a floor for the bladder, uterus and bowels to rest on. The floor of muscles is attached to the pubic bone at the front, and to the base of the spine at the back.

Strong healthy muscles in the pelvic floor support the bladder and bowel, and help in the control of bladder and bowel opening. They are also important during sexual intercourse. Weakness in these muscles may lead to a prolapse of the pelvic organs or to leakage of urine when coughing, sneezing, running or laughing. Weak pelvic floor muscles may also affect the pleasure of sexual intercourse.

The leaking of small amounts of urine resulting from weak muscles is known as stress incontinence. This condition, which can be very distressing, affects one in every four women at some time in their lives.

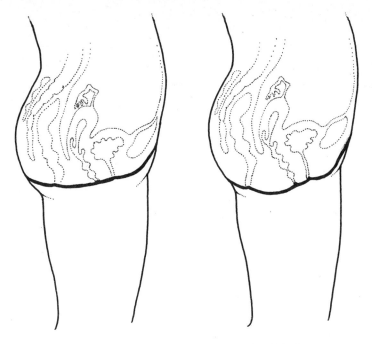

Strong pelvic floor.   **Weak pelvic floor.**

The Pelvic Floor in Pregnancy

The muscles and ligaments in the floor which normally support the abdominal organs may stretch and sag during pregnancy. Two factors may cause this – the weight and size of the baby, and the effect of the hormone progesterone which causes increased stretching of muscles and ligaments.

At the birth, there may be damage to the muscles as the baby's head passes through the pelvis, or by an episiotomy which cuts the muscles, or by the use of forceps. The nerve supply to the muscles may also be damaged. These problems are preventable and treatable. There is no need for women to suffer from them.

Exercises for the Pelvic Floor

1.   Sit in a comfortable position, or lie down with your knees slightly apart. Concentrate on the area where your pelvic floor muscles are. Lift and squeeze at the front as if you were stopping the flow of urine while on the toilet, and lift and squeeze at the back as if you were stopping wind from passing. Hold the lift for as long as you can (at least two seconds). As you get better, increase the time you can hold the squeeze, up to ten

seconds. Rest for an equal number of seconds between each hold. Repeat the squeeze and relaxation as many times as you can – aim for ten squeezes at a time. This should only take up to three minutes – it will be time well spent, and when you have got used to practising this, you can do it while doing something else, for example, reading the newspaper.

2.   Practise the same number of short, fast and strong squeezes. Don't hold your breath, squeeze your buttocks or tighten your abdominal muscles while doing the exercises.

These exercises should be practised as many times as possible every day. Eight times would be ideal and this would still only have taken half an hour. After the baby is born these exercises are most important – it's a good idea to remember to do them when you feed the baby. In fact, they could be done at the same time.

Other ways of protecting the pelvic floor before the birth

1.   Squeeze or hold the pelvic floor muscles before you cough, sneeze or lift anything heavy.

2.   Avoid getting constipated by eating food with plenty of fibre – wholemeal bread, fruit and vegetables and cereals. Try to avoid straining to open your bowels, but if you do have to, then support the muscles between your vagina and anus (front and back) with your fingers.

3.   Try not to get overweight.

4.   Only go to the toilet when your bladder is full.

Problems of Late Pregnancy

Varicose Veins

Women with a tendency to varicose veins may well experience them for the first time during pregnancy. Existing varicose veins may get worse during a pregnancy. The last period of pregnancy is the time when this can become a nuisance. Veins return blood from the body to the heart. Those in the legs are under considerable pressure; in fact, the veins at the ankles experience a pressure of a column of fluid the height of the person acting on quite a small area. Our leg veins are protected from this pressure by valves and by the action of muscles in the legs pumping the blood back up the pressure gradient. In late pregnancy, mothers tend to be less active because of the extra weight they are carrying. The baby in the womb itself makes things worse because it creates congestion in the pelvic area and a further increase in pressure on the veins. The result can be unsightly and painful varicosities which develop as a result of failure of the valves in the veins. Sometimes varicose veins appear in the vulva, and these can be even more uncomfortable.

Prevention and Treatment of Varicose Veins

Understanding the way in which varicose veins are caused leads naturally to ways of preventing and treating them. *Walking* is good for the leg veins because the muscle pump keeps the blood circulating and reduces pressure. *Standing* on the other hand is bad, because the pressure is allowed, but without the countering effect of the muscle pump, so *avoid standing still for more than a few minutes at a time.* Since the problem is caused by pressure from inside the legs, exerting pressure from outside is another way of treating and preventing the problem. *Support stockings or tights* can help in this way. A good combination of exercise and pressure from the outside is *swimming* or *exercise in water.* If you have varicose veins, or a tendency to them, take every opportunity you can of resting in late pregnancy *with the feet elevated.* But remember that you also need to take care of your back. Sitting in a soft chair with the feet up and the back unsupported may well be completely the wrong posture for back care. The best way to rest is therefore on a bed or couch with the feet end raised by about four inches.

Keep the hips, thighs and calves flexible and relaxed by doing the exercises described in this chapter.

Piles

Discomfort and bleeding when having a bowel motion may be caused by piles. These are actually varicose veins around the anus (back passage). Like varicose veins in the legs they tend to get worse in pregnancy, particularly in the last three months when the size of the baby in the womb causes increased pressure in the pelvis. To prevent piles, or to prevent piles getting worse:

– eat lots of fruit, vegetables and whole grain cereals, and drink plenty of fluids to prevent constipation;
– keep up your general fitness by exercising as much as your body will let you;
– do pelvic floor exercises (described earlier in this chapter).

The discomfort of piles can be relieved by soothing ointments such as

Anusol, which is available without prescription from the local chemist. Your family doctor can prescribe other types. *Homoeopathic hammamelis* is said to help piles.

Complications of Pregnancy

Bleeding
Bleeding from the vagina in late pregnancy is potentially serious even if only a small amount, so if this happens consult your midwife or doctor as soon as possible. The two possible serious causes are *placenta praevia* and *antepartum haemorrhage*. Placenta praevia means that the placenta is situated low down in the uterus, covering the cervix partially or wholly so that when labour starts the bleeding may become heavy. If the placenta is wholly covering the cervix, then a caesarean section will be necessary. Antepartum haemorrhage usually means bleeding behind the placenta from some loosening of the placental attachment to the wall of the uterus. A large haemorrhage of this type can compromise the health of both mother and baby and caesarean section is sometimes necessary to deliver the baby safely. Antepartum haemorrhage, also known in this situation as *abruptio placentae*, can show up as abdominal pain with no bleeding.

High Blood Pressure (Hypertension) and Pre-eclampsia
Midwives and doctors rightly fuss about mothers' blood pressure in pregnancy. Blood pressure is expressed as two numbers: xxx/yy. The top number (xxx) is known as *systolic pressure*, which can be thought of as the maximum pressure the heart produces as it pumps blood around the body. The bottom number (yy) is known as *diastolic pressure* and may be likened to the pressure in the heart when it is resting.

In pregnancy, blood pressure changes normally, rising a little from the non-pregnant level at first, falling during the middle of pregnancy and then rising again towards the end. These changes are **normal**. A rise in the diastolic pressure to 95 (the units are millimetres of mercury – mm) or over, however, is considered abnormal. Systolic pressure tends to receive less attention but a rise to 150 or over is also abnormal.

However, a rise in blood pressure **alone** may not be a sign of serious illness or complication. Some people naturally have higher blood pressures from before they were pregnant (*essential hypertension*). This can result in problems if pre-eclampsia occurs in addition. There is an increased risk of pre-eclampsia for women with essential hypertension, so the blood pressure needs careful monitoring and urine testing is done more regularly than for women with 'normal' blood pressures. High blood pressure in the form of essential hypertension without the complication of pre-eclampsia often causes no trouble at all and it may be that no specific treatment is necessary.

Pre-eclampsia

Formerly called *toxaemia of pregnancy*, this has potentially serious consequences for both mother and baby. It is a rise in blood pressure associated with *proteinuria* (protein found in the urine). There may also be *oedema* (swelling of hands and feet) but this is a less important sign.

The consequences of pre-eclampsia for the baby are that the circulation in the placenta is reduced, and thus the baby does not get the nutrition it needs and is less able to deal with waste products. It may become seriously ill and this may be a reason for early delivery, either by induction or by caesarean section. For the mother, the consequences can be equally serious with damage to the kidneys and in very rare but tragic cases, disturbance of blood clotting with haemorrhage, or fits. The very rare but dangerous condition known as *eclampsia* results in convulsions and even coma. The relationship between eclampsia and pre-eclampsia is not really understood.

The consequences of pre-eclampsia are so potentially serious that there is probably, and naturally, a tendency for midwives and doctors to be very cautious about rises in blood pressure in pregnancy. This is particularly the case in hospital antenatal clinics. It is known that anxiety produces a rise in blood pressure and it has been shown in research that anxiety increases in antenatal clinics. To take account of this, some centres researching hypertension in pregnancy have introduced home monitoring of blood pressure for women with hypertension.

Prevention of Pre-eclampsia and Hypertension

At present there is no effective way of preventing pre-eclampsia in a previously healthy mother. For mothers who have had one pregnancy complicated by pre-eclampsia, there is an increased risk in a subsequent pregnancy. Research is still going on into *secondary prevention* of pre-eclampsia (prevention for someone who has already experienced the problem). It seems as though aspirin taken in a low dosage (75mg daily – a 'Junior Aspirin') may be effective in secondary prevention, so there is some hope for such mothers. This is a treatment which should only be taken under medical supervision.

Research is also going on with fish oil and calcium supplements as preventive measures but so far no conclusions have been reached. There is no evidence that bed rest is effective in preventing or treating pre-eclampsia or hypertension in pregnancy.

Some simple measures can prevent a rise in blood pressure, although it must be noted that none of these have been found to prevent pre-eclampsia.

Relaxation seems to be important in nearly every aspect of pregnancy. Perhaps we have to keep emphasising this because of the high levels of stress that seem to be prevalent in our modern society. There is no doubt that doing relaxation exercises, such as the simple ones we described earlier, does produce a fall in blood pressure. It is no use though, doing relaxation exercises for five minutes and lowering blood pressure by 10mm (which is perfectly possible), if this fall in blood pressure only lasts for the time of the exercises and a few minutes afterwards. If we are suffering from stress, then a change in attitude is needed. Exercise can help in this, but won't provide the whole solution if the sources of stress are still present. Remember, stress itself is not a disease. It is part of our natural defence against danger and helps us when we need to produce some extra effort. It can increase heart rate and blood pressure. These sorts of changes can happen when we are under stress, such as approaching the hospital for a check-up. Very often we don't realise how much we are subject to stressful events. Support from family and friends, and confidence in ourselves and feeling good about ourselves in pregnancy can be helpful (see Chapter Two).

Ruth said that she had always had a hatred of seeing the blood pressure machine before she was pregnant and never liked going to the doctors. Perhaps it was surprising that she married Paul, a GP! In her first pregnancy, Ruth felt perfectly well throughout and had no problems until she reached 'term' at 40 weeks. She says, 'I was always conscious of blood pressure. I had no reason to be, but I seemed to have a bee in my bonnet about it. It was normal right up to the last week.'

During the last week, Ruth's blood pressure went up to 150/95. There was no proteinuria, and no other signs of pre-eclampsia, so I agreed with Paul that he would take her blood pressure regularly over the weekend and we would review the situation on Monday if she had not gone into labour.

Nothing had happened by then, so we took the advice of a consultant obstetrician, as Ruth was now ten days overdue with a slightly raised blood pressure. He reassured us all that we could simply watch and wait.

By Wednesday, however, Ruth's blood pressure had gone up to 160/105, and now she had proteinuria. She had to go to hospital, where she was given a prostin pessary to try to start labour, and a drip with drugs to control the blood pressure. As the prostin didn't work, she was given another drip with syntocinon to start contractions, and her waters were broken. She says, 'I was totally wired up, with a monitor as well. All I could do was look at the clock on the wall. The syntocinon caused painful, rapid contractions which were quite severe.' She was given an epidural which made her more comfortable and helped to control the blood pressure. She felt safe because 'I had a midwife to myself all the time, so I had quite a lot of attention.' At one point there was some anxiety about the monitor trace and a registrar was called. He decided to perform a caesarean section. Ruth continues, 'At this point Paul stepped in. He asked if the registrar was sure this was the right thing to do.' The registrar called his boss, the consultant, who looked at the monitor and took a fetal blood sample. It was fine. He decided to watch and wait for a further three hours. Ruth says, 'I thought, "Oh, no! Another three hours; I can't lie in this position for another three hours," but after another hour, I felt the head pushing down. Paul and the midwife looked at me as if I was joking. The midwife checked and said yes, the head was there! They could only let me push for half an hour because of the blood pressure. Paul was a great help at this time.' Catherine was born safe and sound half an hour later with no other intervention needed.

This story, as well as illustrating some of the problems for women with high blood pressure, shows how a husband can help his wife to assert herself when very vulnerable. Paul had the advantage of being a doctor, but any husband or partner could have made the same intervention to the registrar who wanted to do a caesarean. He merely politely asked a question, which produced a good result. Ruth says that at the time she actually wanted to have a caesarean to get it all over with, but that she was very glad she didn't and that Paul had helped her in this way.

Twins

By this stage of a pregnancy, a mother should know if she is carrying twins. Twin pregnancies can become complicated during the last three months.

There is a greater risk of pre-eclampsia and of premature labour. The extra weight and size of the babies can make the mother feel more tired and have more back problems. For this reason, extra rest is usually necessary and some obstetricians regularly offer mothers with twins hospital admission for rest in the last month, or earlier. We would advise mothers with twins to have a consultant unit birth because of the possible complications of the birth itself as well as the possible complications of late pregnancy.

The main problems with birth for twins are:

- the babies tend to be small and are often born prematurely. Small babies and premature babies may need paediatric care in a Special Care Baby Unit immediately after birth and perhaps until they are safe to be cared for by the mother alone;
- the breech presentation is more common for one or both twins and so are other 'malpresentations' such as a transverse lie which often requires caesarean section;
- the second twin tends to be more stressed by the birth, having experienced contractions for longer.

The principles of preparation for birth remain the same, though. Most mothers of twins tell us that the labour itself is usually not too long or more uncomfortable than with single pregnancies and this seems to fit with our own observations. Be prepared, though, for more intervention in the birth because of the greater risk of fetal distress and of malpresentation.

Dawn had one baby, Belinda, aged one year when she became pregnant again. She was very distressed to find that she was carrying twins, which we confirmed for her by a scan. Once she got over the shock, she began to feel better about carrying two babies and was able to prepare for the hard work she knew was ahead of her. She describes her pregnancy:

'You could feel them both moving but I couldn't tell which was which until later when they explained to me where they were lying. I felt really sick. It felt totally different from Belinda. I felt more run down, I was more tired, really shattered. I wanted to eat more. Near the end I couldn't sleep. I couldn't lie down comfortably. I had to prop myself up with pillows. Even sitting was uncomfortable. I had to sit with my legs apart and put cushions behind my back. Massaging myself with oils helped a bit; it eased the pain in my belly. It used to hurt under the ribs.'

Dawn felt that she could have been better prepared for the birth:

'My waters broke and I went into labour. It was normal at first, then Heather came out and it started all over again. That was the worst part, waiting for it to start all over again. I was all right till I walked into the labour ward. All the machines, you just don't expect it, and all the people there. There seemed to be loads of people. No one had explained that, I wasn't prepared for it: the drip, the people, the monitor. I found it all a bit scary. I had one doctor asking me lots of questions, another putting up a drip and another taking blood from me. They were nice, but nobody had explained what would happen. Jessica (the second twin) was a breech. They put my legs up in stirrups. She was stuck. The doctor put his hand in and just pulled her out. She didn't breathe at first and I was a bit worried but she was all right in the end. I'd been told that you had to stay in for ten days afterwards, but I only stayed for three, so that was better.'

The Breech Position

A baby is said to be a 'breech' when its bottom or feet are presenting to the cervix (conversely the head will be up at the top of the uterus). Breech births are more complicated than those (the majority) where the head comes first. There is an increasing tendency for caesarean sections to be performed routinely for breech births.

BREECH=CAESAREAN?

Evidence There is at present no evidence to support this practice. There is, however, a growing body of evidence about the value of *external cephalic version* for breech presentation.

External Cephalic Version is an old technique which involves rotating the breech baby around in the uterus by manipulation through the mother's abdominal wall. This can be done quite gently by an experienced person. The risks to mother and baby are almost negligible and the benefits considerable since caesarean section may be avoided.

EXTERNAL CEPHALIC VERSION

Evidence The best time to do ECV is at term, but it should certainly not be done before 37 weeks, firstly because spontaneous rotation to the cephalic (head down) position may occur, and secondly, because there is less chance of the baby reverting to its old position. Some obstetricians give drugs to relax the uterus before doing the version. The evidence is that this is unnecessary unless there has already been an unsuccessful attempt to turn the baby without the use of drugs.

Other methods of encouraging a breech baby to turn

There is some evidence that practising certain postures regularly each day may encourage the baby to turn.

POSTURE

Evidence The numbers of cases in research so far have not been enough to be sure if these methods really work.
Opinion We think that trying this can do no harm so if you have a breech baby in the last month of pregnancy, why not give it a try?

Put a large cushion or two on the floor and lie down with your hips on the cushions and your head on the floor, so that your pelvis is higher than your head. Put a small cushion or pillow under your head if you need it. In this position, the baby will drop away from the pelvis and begin to move. Relax and take deep breaths. Stay in this position for 10 to 15 minutes each day. Mothers tell us that they talk to their babies when doing this, and tell them to turn. We think that this sort of communication between mother and baby can only be good. Who knows, it may help to produce the desired result! A little gentle massage on the tummy with some oil can do no harm either and helps the communication process.

Some homoeopathic remedies are claimed to assist in turning a breech baby. We feel that for this it would be wise to consult a qualified and experienced homoeopath or homoeopathic doctor. Acupuncture is also said to help.

Contractions

Contractions occur in the uterus almost from the beginning of pregnancy. They tend to become more apparent towards the end and can be painful and alarming. These contractions, which occur irregularly, are called Braxton–Hicks contractions and are normal. They don't mean the start of premature labour or that anything is wrong. However, if you're unsure about whether contractions are this type, or the 'real thing', don't be afraid to get in touch with your midwife or doctor for reassurance.

Medical Problems in Pregnancy

Asthma

This need not be a problem in pregnancy or in labour if it is well controlled using modern inhalers. The inhalers used for asthma are known as *preventers* and *relievers*. These do what their names suggest. Preventers are anti-inflammatory drugs which are taken regularly, every day, to prevent attacks of asthma. They are either steroids (Beclamethasone or Becotide being the most commonly used) or Disodium Cromoglycate (intal). Relievers act on the small air tubes in the lungs, to dilate them when they are narrowed by an attack of asthma. Relievers are drugs like Salbutamol (Ventolin).

The beauty of inhalers is that large concentrations of drug get into the lungs where they are needed, but only very small amounts get into the bloodstream. This means that only very minute amounts of inhaled drugs for asthma can cross the placenta to the baby. **It is most important that mothers who suffer from asthma continue to use their inhalers in pregnancy**. There is no evidence of any effects on the baby from inhaled asthma drugs. Any theoretical effect from the very small amount of drug which crosses the placenta should be minimal.

In late pregnancy, the size of the baby and uterus and the restriction of movement of the diaphragm may affect breathing capacity. This may also be the case in labour, when an asthma attack would be a nuisance at least, so in preparing for labour, asthmatic mothers would be advised to make sure their asthma control is the best it can possibly be. Have your inhalers with you when you go into labour. If in doubt, seek advice from your doctor. Mothers who regularly have to take steroids by mouth for their asthma (the most commonly used is Prednisolone) ought to have specialist care, both for their asthma and for their pregnancy and labour.

Diabetes

This causes particular problems in pregnancy, both for mother and baby. The pregnancy may alter the mother's need for insulin and the daily dose may need to be altered to accommodate this. It may be necessary to give insulin more frequently than the usual twice daily regime. Diabetic mothers have a greater risk of hypertension (high blood pressure) in pregnancy. Going back to early pregnancy, hypoglycaemia (blood sugar too low) may be a problem because of the unstable situation produced by the pregnancy and because of vomiting or loss of appetite, which some women experience at this time. If this happens, mothers should not use glucose or sugar when they feel a 'hypo' coming on. Instead, milk or a light snack should be taken. This is because it has been found that in early pregnancy, diabetic mothers naturally tend to overtreat their hypoglycaemic attacks and cause their blood sugar levels to be too high. If the mother's blood sugar is too high, this can affect the baby, causing oedema or fluid retention, affecting the baby's kidneys.

There is also an association of diabetes with larger babies. For this reason and those stated above, diabetic mothers need very careful monitoring during pregnancy and labour, and usually need specialist care, both for their diabetes and for the pregnancy. Most hospitals have a close liaison between the obstetricians and the diabetic specialists for the care of diabetic mothers. There has been a tendency for diabetic mothers to be delivered before term to avoid complications of diabetes for the baby.

DIABETES=EARLY DELIVERY?

Evidence This was an incorrect policy and it is now recommended that diabetic mothers should go to full term unless there are obstetric reasons for intervening to deliver the baby early.

Diabetic mothers also have a greater risk of having a caesarean section although there is no evidence that this is advisable because of the diabetes itself. The evidence shows that caesarean section should be kept for obstetric indications.

We advise diabetic mothers, just as we advise non-diabetic mothers, to ask questions about decisions made about their care. Don't be satisfied with, 'It's for the good of the baby.' If you are faced with a decision, such as a caesarean, which you are not sure about, ask *what evidence* there is to support this decision. There may well be a perfectly good reason for the advice you are given, but you will feel more in control and more satisfied with your care if you understand why things are being done.

There is a condition of temporary diabetes in pregnancy – 'gestational diabetes' – which is uncovered when testing the urine and sugar is found. Although there is only a very slight increase in risk to the baby when this occurs, which is mainly because of a tendency to an increase in size, there is no evidence that any form of treatment of this condition is effective. Much anxiety is caused by telling women that they have some form of diabetes, which could be dispelled by full explanation. The glucose found in the urine of such women always disappears after the birth.

Epilepsy

There are two difficulties for a mother with epilepsy. First, the drugs used to control her fits may cause some harm to the baby. Phenytoin (Epanutin), Carbamazepine (Tegretol) and Sodium Valproate (Epilim), are the three most commonly used drugs. There are small differences between them, but the most important finding for mothers taking them is that 5% to 10% of babies born to mothers taking these drugs have congenital abnormalities involving the face, fingers and toes. Hare lip and cleft palate are examples of these.

Secondly, the pregnancy may cause an increase in the tendency to fits. This may be because of changes in the mother's metabolism affecting levels of the drugs used to control the epilepsy. The consequences of a fit are potentially dangerous to both mother and baby, so the balance lies with continuing the medication throughout pregnancy. There is a higher risk of congenital abnormalities for mothers using more than one drug to control their epilepsy but there are also risks of provoking a fit in changing medication, so this is best done while planning to be pregnant (see Chapter One).

Although these drugs are found in breast milk, the levels are not sufficient to cause any effect in the babies, so mothers taking these drugs may breast feed safely.

Preparing for the Baby

Shopping

There is very considerable marketing pressure on mothers to buy equipment for their babies. A new baby actually has very few needs, especially in terms of equipment, so there is no need to rush into expensive purchases. We've noticed that many of the free books on pregnancy, that are handed out in antenatal clinics and parentcraft classes, carry advertisements for equipment and even articles recommending certain types of equipment. We recommend mothers to be cautious in reading these, and to remember that the books are free because of the advertising they carry. Even the two free booklets produced by the Royal College of Midwives ('Pregnancy' and 'Babycare') and the Royal College of General Practitioners ('Emma's Diary') contain heavy advertising for equipment and although both of these publications promote breast feeding strongly, they both have several large and prominent advertisements for bottle milk inside.

The new baby will need:

– some clothes;
– somewhere to sleep;
– some nappies;
– somewhere to wash;
– if not breastfed, some equipment for feeding (see Chapter Eight);

and perhaps not immediately:

– some means for you to transport them when outside the home – a pram or pushchair.

Clothes

Babies grow very rapidly and soon become too big for first-size clothes, so get only the minimum number. Loose-fitting clothes allow for growth and make dressing easier. Stretch suits ('babygrows') are the most practical clothes, and can be used in the day and the night. Babies do not control their body temperatures well at first, so they must not be too hot because of too many clothes or too cold. The most heat loss comes from a baby's head so hats are important. The safest clothes are the simplest, without strings that might fasten tightly around the neck, or loose parts that might find their way into the mouth.

Shopping List for Clothes

◆ Four cotton vests
◆ Three or four stretch suits ('babygrows')

- Two cardigans
- Two or three pairs of socks or bootees
- One or two pairs of mittens
- One or two woolly hats
- Two or three blankets

Sleeping

The baby won't need a cot until he or she is three or four months old. A carrycot is the most practical first bed. It is portable, both indoors and out, and can be anchored to the back seat of a car and used as a pram if it has a chassis with wheels. Carrycots should conform to British Standard BS 3881 for safety.

Alternatives are Moses baskets and cribs, which are much more decorative, but less practical. There are no safety standards for these.

Safety

- Never put a pillow in the baby's cot.
- Always put your baby to sleep lying on the back or side, **never** face down.

COT DEATH

Evidence There is overwhelming evidence, from large studies in New Zealand and the UK, that putting the baby to sleep on the back or side, and never face down, prevents the tragedy of cot death.

Another very important factor in cot death is smoking. Cot death is three times more common for babies whose parents smoke.

- If you put the carrycot in the car, you should use a carrycot car restraint fitted to the back seat (BSAU 186A). There has been much in the news about baby seats in cars, and these should be chosen with great care.
- It is dangerous to carry a baby in the front passenger seat if a passenger airbag has been fitted.
- It is dangerous to hold a baby in your arms in the car because, in an accident, the baby could be thrown out of your arms and become seriously injured.

Nappies

The choice is between disposable nappies and cloth (terry) nappies. Our impression is that the introduction of disposables has reduced the incidence of nappy rash, but we don't have research evidence for this observation. Disposables are easier to use and require less work and equipment, but are more expensive in the long term and are becoming a problem in the environment because they do not decompose readily. However, if other factors are considered in the cost, such as mother's time spent washing, electricity to heat the water and washing powder, perhaps the cost is not much different from terry nappies.

Disposables are now subtly different for boys and girls. Terry nappies need a larger initial outlay but are, of course, re-usable. They need washing and sterilising. They can be used with waterproof pants.

Shopping List for Disposable Nappies

- One pack of newborn-size disposable nappies
- One pack of nappy sacks
- One pot of cream (Sudocrem)

Shopping List for Terry Nappies

- 24 terry nappies
- Nappy liners
- Two pairs of waterproof pants
- Two nappy buckets (ordinary buckets with lids will do)
- Sanitising fluid or powder (Nappisan)
- Safety pins

A changing mat is also useful, but not absolutely essential.

Bathing

A plastic oval or rectangular bowl is a perfectly good baby bath for the first three months, after which babies can be bathed in the family bath. Special baby baths are more expensive. There are many types and accessories, none of which seem to us to have any advantages. Some soft towels will be needed, and some cotton wool.

CHAPTER SEVEN

GIVING BIRTH

....

The Beginning of Labour

There are two signs that labour is starting – contractions which are regular and strong, and the waters breaking. Some mothers may have a 'show', the passage of a small amount of blood and mucus a few days before labour starts. This is perfectly normal, but larger amounts of blood or persistent bleeding need urgent attention from a midwife or doctor.

Contractions can occur throughout pregnancy, and can be painful especially towards the end of pregnancy, so sometimes mothers experiencing these can be unsure about whether they are in labour. The best rule is if you're unsure, ask your midwife or doctor. Even they may be unsure! It is a regular occurrence that we, as doctors and midwives, talk about, when mothers come into hospital, thinking they are in labour, to be told they are not and sent home, only to reappear half an hour later with strong contractions and almost ready to give birth. If the waters break, then it is definitely time to contact a midwife or doctor. Quite often though, the waters don't break until later in labour or even just before the baby is born.

We advise our mothers that babies born in taxis and buses and in the car on the way to hospital are really very rare. Most mothers have plenty of time, when labour starts, to prepare themselves, get things ready, have a cup of tea, ring husband or partner or whoever they would like to be at the birth, ring the midwife and/or the doctor and make their arrangements to give birth either at home or in hospital. Labours lasting less than an hour are most unusual and most last for several hours. So, when labour starts, try to remember and practise all the parts of your preparation. Who will be with you? How will you relax? What sort of pain relief will you use? What things would you like around you? What music? Take your time, get these things organised in your own mind first, and then in practise. If it's a first baby and you are going to hospital, it may take quite a long time for it to be born, and you may have to spend some hours there not doing very much, so don't hurry, and be prepared.

The First Stage of Labour

Every mother is different from every other mother. Each baby is different from every other. Every pregnancy is different from all other pregnancies and every labour is different from all other labours. This is our observation from our involvement in several hundred births. Textbooks describe a certain pattern, midwives and doctors have certain expectations, but few mothers seem to conform to what is expected. Contractions vary in timing and intensity. The site and nature of the pain and its strength vary for each mother and for each birth. The way labour starts (the beginning of the first stage) is very variable.

It is the baby who decides when labour starts. Changes in the baby's adrenal gland lead to secretion of a hormone which probably triggers the whole process. The uterus, which has been contracting, sometimes unnoticed, throughout pregnancy, now begins to contract regularly with painful contractions, perhaps every 20 minutes. The frequency of the contractions increases to every five minutes, and the intensity of the pain with each contraction builds up as labour progresses.

As the contractions increase, the cervix, or neck of the womb is taken up so that it becomes closely applied to the baby's head. The cervix then begins to open up or *dilate*. Hospital midwives and doctors will define the beginning of labour as the point when the cervix begins to dilate. This results, as we have illustrated above, in some women being told that they are not in labour because the cervix is not dilated. Our experience is that many of these mothers know that they are in labour and tell us afterwards that they certainly were, even though there was no cervical dilatation.

The first stage ends when the cervix is fully dilated – open sufficiently to allow the baby to be born. The first stage is very variable in length and can last up to 24 hours or more without intervention to hasten the process. It could be as little as an hour or even less, but these are the extremes.

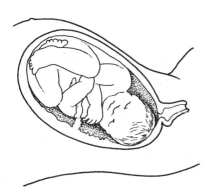 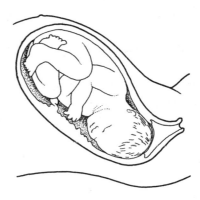

The early first stage.

The late first stage with the cervix dilated.

What to do in the First Stage

Again, every labour is unique. For most mothers, the first stage will last for several hours, so unless you live in a remote place, away from professional help, or have a history of rapid labour, or some complication of pregnancy which requires specialist help, our advice is that when labour starts, take your time. If you are having a hospital birth, you may have to spend several hours in the ward; this time may seem to pass very slowly, so don't hurry in to the hospital unless you have to.

Take time to prepare yourself, carry on for as long as possible with whatever you were doing or whatever you want to do in the day. Have a bath, have a cup of tea or a snack, gather your things around you, tell everyone who you want to know what is happening, then wait a little longer! Don't forget your husband, partner or supporter will also have to spend long hours with you in labour, and may need fortifying with a snack at the beginning. If in doubt about whether to go to the hospital or not, call a midwife or your family doctor. Don't hurry and don't panic.

Staying in Control

When a mother goes into hospital, and to a lesser extent when she calls a midwife or doctor to attend her birth at home, there is a sense in which she is submitting to control by someone else. Although hospital staff certainly don't intend this to be the case, the very nature of a large hospital is that it is a busy, bewildering environment, and mothers can find themselves being told to do this, go there, breathe like this . . . Most mothers want to feel in command of themselves. A few prefer to have someone else in charge when they are in labour, but our experience is that the vast majority resent being ordered about and feel much more comfortable when they are in control of themselves and their own labour. It can be very difficult to keep this sense of control, especially when in the second stage of labour, but fortunately for mothers, most will have a husband, partner or supporter with them, who they can brief to act for them if they find they are being forced to do something they don't want to do or don't understand.

We encourage our mothers and their partners to be assertive. This means standing up for yourself politely but firmly. Preparation for birth is the key to assertiveness during labour. It's too late to change habits when the contractions start, and certainly not possible to change your personality. We described some simple exercises in assertiveness in Chapter Two.

Jinni had a normal pregnancy but went into the forty-second week of pregnancy. By now she was feeling, as many mothers do, pretty fed-up. She developed mild hypertension, her blood pressure being slightly raised, though without any sign of pre-eclampsia, and we agreed together that she should be transferred to consultant care for induction of labour. She describes the experience: 'Up until the birth it was fine, because then it was discussed with you at length and agreed, but once I went into hospital I felt like I had been abandoned somehow, although I had a very nice midwife there. But at the time I was very frightened.' Despite the fear, she remembered some of the things we had discussed in the group meetings and was able to regain control of herself and assert herself:

'The doctor who came to do the induction never introduced himself. I had to ask who he was. He could have been anybody off the street wearing a white coat. That was something we learned at antenatal, to ask and not to be pushed around.'

Positions for the First Stage

Many people carry in their minds the traditional picture of a woman in labour, which has only really been prevalent in twentieth-century western society. This picture has the mother lying in or on a bed, on her back. This is the worst possible position for labour, both for mother and baby for several reasons, the most obvious being anatomy. To be born from this position, the baby has actually to travel upwards through the mother's pelvis, against gravity. This is also the worst position for the action of the uterus and for the mother to push in the second stage.

An upright posture throughout labour, but especially in the first stage, does result in shorter labour.

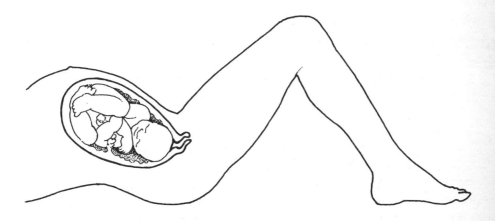

The mechanical disadvantage of lying down in labour.

UPRIGHT=SHORTER LABOUR?

Evidence from research confirms this and also shows that women who remain upright during the first stage require less pain-relieving drugs than those who lie down. Research also shows that lying on her back reduces the output of blood from the mother's heart and also reduces the flow of blood through the uterus and placenta; therefore, there may be theoretical effects on the baby.

Research studies have not, however, shown that this theoretical effect is translated into actual harm to the baby from the mother lying on her back.

Evidence is that contractions are more efficient when mothers are upright during the first stage. All this evidence therefore should convince mothers that it is best to stay upright for as much as possible during the first stage of labour.

How to keep the Best Position in the First Stage

- ◆ Use people, pillows or furniture to give support.
- ◆ Rocking the pelvis from side to side is very comforting and probably helps the baby to descend.
- ◆ Bending the knees helps rocking and helps to avoid tiredness in the legs.
- ◆ Keep the feet apart to give a wide base for support.
- ◆ Partners can be helpful – a dancing position is both comfortable and comforting.
- ◆ Creative use of furniture, pillows and other objects can help give support – these can be noted before labour (see above).
- ◆ An asymmetrical position can be helpful.

Breathing

We all know how relaxing a deep breath and a sigh can be – the sigh of relief. Most relaxation exercises include methods that involve breathing techniques. Simply concentrating on breathing during labour can help mothers to relax and to relieve some of the discomfort of labour.

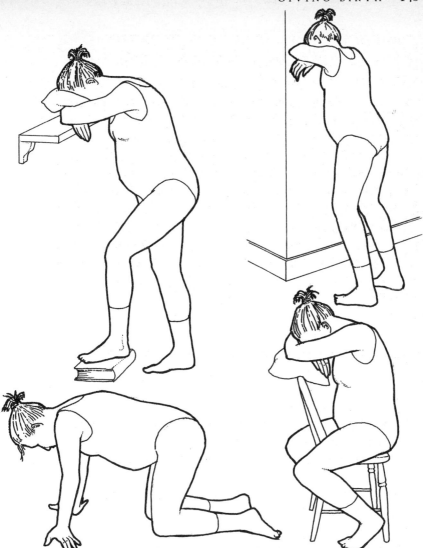

Positions for labour in the first stage.

A Simple Breathing Exercise for the First Stage

Close the eyes and let your breath in, picture the breath travelling down the backbone, over the baby and down to the floor.

Allow the shoulders, back and face to soften with each *outbreath*. Let the arms and back and face feel heavier and heavier each time you breathe out.

This trick takes only a minute and can be used any time, in moments of panic, during contractions or during times of rest. During contractions, find something to support you, a chair or even just a wall to lean against, and then breathe . . .

Food During the First Stage

There is a natural tendency for women in labour not to want to eat. It's certainly not a good idea to eat large meals or indigestible food, but labour is a big drain on energy resources and can last for a long time, therefore it is a good plan to replenish energy supplies from time to time. The best things to eat and drink are high-energy foods – carbohydrates, but foods that are light and easily digestible. Cereals, fruit juices, toast and jam or honey – in fact, breakfast foods, which tend to be high-energy foods to start the day.

When labour starts, it may be a good idea if the body says it feels like it, to eat a light meal of bread and soup for example, or an egg, or yoghurt. Whatever feels best is often best. As labour progresses, have some high-energy fruit drinks handy to keep up energy stores. For hospital births, you'll have to bring in the foods and drinks you want to use, and get your partner to supply them to you. Many hospitals have a policy of not permitting food to be eaten during labour. The reason for this is to prevent aspiration of stomach contents into the lungs. This is a potentially serious event but the likelihood of it happening is extremely small and is almost always associated with general anaesthesia.

FOOD DURING LABOUR

Evidence There is no good reason for complete restriction of food and drink during labour.

Hospitals are increasingly adopting a policy of allowing the sort of light high-energy foods described above. If your hospital is a restrictive one, then it may be best to use the sort of high-energy drinks that marathon runners use to maintain your energy levels.

Your Environment for Labour

In the last chapter we described how to prepare for labour in choice of place, people and position. When in labour, all the preparation can be put into practice. We keep emphasising that labour is very individual and it must be said at this stage, that all the plans and preparation may go out of the window when labour actually starts! Sometimes, to take a relatively trivial example, mothers decide in preparation that they would like their favourite music playing during the first stage, but when it comes to the crunch, they find they actually want to curl up and be quiet and undisturbed. Some like someone to talk to and keep chatting throughout, others want to be isolated and go 'within themselves' communicating only for the essentials. Be prepared to experience these feelings and to change what you had prepared, following your natural instincts. The most important thing is to be able to tell your attendants either directly or through your partner, just what it is that you want and how you would like to be treated. If something is annoying you, say so. In particular, if you can't get on with one of the people attending you, midwife or doctor, say so as politely as you can. It's your right to have someone else to look after you.

LABOUR ATTENDANTS

Evidence Research shows that the influence of a trusted attendant on the outcome of labour is very strong.

Let's assume though, that the preparation was right: the place is right, the right people are with you and you are able to adopt the best and most comfortable position that you have practised. Now is the time for your partner to put on the music you want, or to create quiet and dim lighting if that's what makes you feel more comfortable. These conditions that constitute your present environment will be the best for encouraging efficient contractions of the uterus, which will take up the cervix and cause it to open (dilate) to allow the birth of the baby.

Breaking the Waters (Rupturing the Membranes, ARM)

This is a procedure that has become increasingly common during labour. Many midwives do it as a routine, believing that it will shorten the labour. An ARM is done in exactly the same way as it is used to induce labour. The plastic 'amnihook' is introduced into the vagina and guided by hand onto the membranes overlying the baby's head. A hole is made in the membranes with the implement. We do not perform this procedure routinely for our mothers.

ARM

Opinion We think that there is no good reason to interfere by doing an ARM in most labours. Most mothers certainly want labour to be as short as possible, but we are not convinced that shortening labour artificially is desirable. There is a risk of introducing infection by doing an ARM. Breaking the membranes removes their function as extra protection for the cord and the baby's head during the final stages of labour. When an ARM seems to accelerate labour, it is likely that the membranes would have broken on their own.

Evidence There is little research evidence about performing an ARM in labour either in favour or against. The only reliable finding is that an early ARM does shorten labour by, on average, 60 to 120 minutes. There is no convincing evidence that ARM causes either beneficial or harmful effects on the baby.

Our advice is, if asked whether or not the membranes should be ruptured, ask why the person concerned thinks that this will help.

Pain Relief

All the measures we discussed above and in the previous chapter: people, place and position; relaxation, breathing and hypnosis, can help to relieve pain in labour. For some mothers, these are all that are required. TENS may be the next step and we have certainly seen many mothers use nothing else except a TENS machine during labour. Mothers using TENS should preferably have practised with the machine in the weeks before labour starts and their partners should also be familiar with it so that they can help by putting the electrodes in the correct place, and re-positioning them, if necessary. As labour progresses, it may be necessary to turn up the 'gain' on the machine, to strengthen the impulse it provides to give a greater effect. A partner may be able to remind the mother of this, and to help her with the controls of the machine.

Alternatively, the birthing pool may supply all the pain relief needs for some mothers.

Everyone experiences pain differently and while some mothers may not require any additional pain relief, others need the help of pharmaceutical analgesics.

'Gas and Air' (Entonox)

This is a 50–50 mixture of oxygen and nitrous oxide which the mother inhales through a mask. It has the advantages that the mother herself can control the use of the gas, and that the effects wear off quickly and do not harm the baby. It does not affect the efficiency of the contractions or the ability to bear down or push in the second stage. The disadvantages are that it is a relatively weak pain killer, is mildly sedative and its side effects are nausea and vomiting. Some women find it very helpful.

Pethidine and other Analgesics given by injection

Pethidine is a drug similar to morphine in its action. It is a strong analgesic (pain killer). It has an effect similar to morphine which can make the mother oblivious to the passage of time and it also has a relaxing effect on the cervix and can shorten labour, but has the disadvantage that it is heavily sedative and can reduce a mother's sense of being in control of herself and her birth. Its other side effects include nausea and vomiting. It causes respiratory depression for the baby – that means it depresses the baby's ability to breathe. This effect can be reversed by an injection of the 'antidote' naloxone being given to the baby after birth. A drug similar to Pethidine in strength of analgesic effect, but with fewer side effects, is Meptazinol, which is used surprisingly little in hospital obstetric practice.

The depressing effect on the baby's breathing is increased if Pethidine is given to a mother who has also taken barbiturates and this could be very dangerous to the baby.

It is wise not to have Pethidine if the birth is likely to occur soon, again because of the respiratory depressant effect.

Gillian used 'gas and air', TENS and had an injection of Pethidine during the birth of Natalie, her first baby. She says, 'I couldn't cope with the gas and air. I didn't feel as if I was in control. The room kept spinning round and it made me cough. The TENS machine was good.

'To be honest, things were going very slow and although I was having contractions every ten minutes or so, they didn't last more than 30 seconds. They kept asking if I wanted Pethidine. I was told I could have two injections and they would last about two hours. I thought I was only two centimetres, so I had better wait until the contractions got worse and I really needed the injection. When the waters broke, there was lots of Meconium. They gave me the Pethidine then, but everything happened very quickly after that. I didn't feel any pain then, so I assume it was the Pethidine that made it OK.

'When Natalie came out she didn't cry or anything and she was very dopey. She had a very low Apgar Score, so I think that was due to the Pethidine.'

Fiona had an injection of Pethidine during the birth of her second baby, Simon. She says, 'I think I was getting a bit anxious, so I think they gave it to me to calm me down a bit. I don't think I had the full effect because it was quite late on when they gave it to me. I think it relieved some of the pain but not all of it. I didn't get out of control and I didn't feel drowsy. I think with the second one you're more het up because you know what's coming.'

Clare had a very bad experience with Pethidine in the birth of her first baby, Robbie. Labour was slow because, as it turned out, Robbie was in the 'O-P' position: he was born looking up rather than down. The midwife asked Clare if she wanted some Pethidine. Clare continues the story: 'I said, "I don't really want it at the moment." She said, "It will be a long night." She came again half an hour later and asked again. I looked at Peter (Clare's partner) and asked him what he thought. She said, "Why are you asking him?" She implied that I would be doing myself a favour if I had the injection, so I gave in, but afterwards I wished I hadn't. There was no difference, it wasn't like instant pain relief. My contractions seemed to come all together and then I had a rest for about 20 minutes, then they would come again. I never had the urge to push. I went "pathetic", my thinking was blurred. When she was saying "push", I lost any conviction to do anything myself. I just sort of lay there, hoping it would come out. It made me very thirsty as well. I felt as though I had had too much to drink, and was not quite with what was going on. I didn't feel like that the second time.'

Clare's second baby, Benjamin, was also 'O-P', but this time she refused the Pethidine and got into the all-fours position, which she says was more effective in relieving the pain. She felt much more in control during the birth of Benjamin.

These two mothers had different experiences with Pethidine. Fiona's was more positive than Clare's, but they have one thing in common: both were given the drug without really giving informed consent. Even with the sort of preparation for assertiveness that we have discussed in Chapter Two, it can be very difficult to make your wishes known when you are vulnerable, having strong contractions. Like Clare's partner, Peter, many a husband or partner may find it difficult to help because he sees someone he loves in distress.

Epidural and Spinal Anaesthesia

These are both techniques for giving almost total pain relief to the lower half of the body by means of an injection of anaesthetic into the spine to numb the nerves which join the spinal cord, transmitting the feeling of pain to the brain. The advantages are that labour can be virtually pain-free; for someone with high blood pressure, the anaesthetic reduces the pressure; and if caesarean section is necessary then this can be done by simply topping up the anaesthetic through a cannula already in place. Many women find the absence of pain in labour a wonderful experience.

An anaesthetist is needed to give the epidural. A needle is inserted between the bones of the spine, then a plastic tube is fed down the needle to the fluid surrounding the nerves of the spinal cord. The needle is removed and the tube is left in place. Anaesthetic is injected down the tube and takes effect in about 15 minutes. The anaesthetic can be topped up from time to time as needed during labour.

The disadvantages for women using epidural or spinal anaesthesia are that labour tends to be longer; there is complete inability to feel or use the legs; pushing is less efficient in the second stage; and statistically there is a greater likelihood of instrumental delivery – by ventouse, forceps or caesarean section. A catheter (tube) into the bladder is usually necessary after the birth because there may be no sensation of wanting to pass urine. A recent advance in technology is the 'mobile epidural' which allows women in labour to be up and about and not to need catheterisation. This technique has not yet been fully evaluated by research and it is not known whether the pain relief is as effective as with a standard epidural. It is not yet widely available.

In our experience, the disadvantages of epidurals and spinals are rarely explained to mothers fully, especially the risk of a further complication found in research, which is that 30% of women having epidural or spinal anaesthesia in labour develop chronic back pain after the birth. This pain can be lifelong in some cases and there is little effective treatment for it. Another complication is headache, which usually gets better after a few days, but sometimes persists for weeks and, rarely, months after the birth.

Jinni, who we met earlier, eventually had an epidural for her first birth. She said that the pain relief did not work completely, but it 'made it bearable.' Oliver was born after 14 hours in labour. She planned to have an epidural for the second time, but this time her labour was much quicker and there was no time to give the epidural. Imogen was born after three hours. Jinni says, 'Recovery was much quicker without the epidural. My back ached every time I gave Oliver a bath, but I had no problems with Imogen. This time the birth was completely bearable and three hours seemed a very short time.'

Ruth, who had pre-eclampsia (Chapter Six), had a good experience with her epidural. 'The epidural worked. I had no after effects at all. It was perfect. It was just right because it took away the pain, but I still had a sensation at the end because it was just beginning to wear off.'

She did have a few problems, however. 'I was really wired up: I had two drips, a catheter, the epidural and a monitor. The worst thing about it was the number of wires. When my waters broke, I wanted to go to the toilet and it was a major operation to get me off the bed.'

Using the Birthing Pool – Hydrotherapy and 'Water Birth'

Water can be useful as a means of relaxation and getting pain relief in labour. It can also be a good environment in which to give birth. The birthing pool can be used either for pain relief in the first stage with the mother getting out as she enters the second stage and the baby being born on 'dry land', or the baby can be born in the water.

Our practice has a birthing pool, which was purchased with the aid of a local charity. This pool is used by our mothers, either in the GP unit of the local hospital, or in their homes. We make no charge for use of the pool but ask the mothers to arrange transport of it to wherever they are going to use it. The pool is portable and consists of four fibreglass sections which, when bolted together, make an oval pool. A thick polythene liner is then fitted into the pool. Each mother therefore has her own inner liner which is only used once and then discarded – although one father said he would make a garden pond out of his. The pool is filled with hot and cold water from a garden hose. The volume of water in the pool is nearly 200 gallons. This volume of water maintains its temperature well but to assist this there is a thermal cover, which is also nice for the mother to hide under. A thermometer is used to keep the temperature steady by topping up with warm water, as necessary. The temperature should be about body temperature, 37.4° Celsius.

The advantages of using the birthing pool are:

Water is naturally relaxing to all of us. When we get home from work or reach the end of a long, hard day, a natural reaction is to subside into a nice, warm bath. As we get into the bath, we let out a great sigh of relief. In the birthing pool, a mother can relax, float and adopt any comfortable position. The weight of her body is partly supported by the water.

But the water does more than just provide relaxation, it seems to provide pain relief in itself. In some way, the water in a bath probably stimulates our naturally occurring pain killing, morphine-like substances, endorphins and relieves our aching limbs. So it seems to be in labour.

A third advantage of the birthing pool is that it provides a sheltered environment for the woman in labour into which she can retreat if she wishes to be quiet and alone. Many women do feel this way and resent interference with their privacy in labour. The water is a barrier against the hands of interfering doctors and midwives and, for that matter, any other unwanted supporters. Whenever we state this opinion in lectures to midwives or doctors, there are always gasps. Is it not 'unsafe' to be unable to use one's hands to examine a woman in labour? There is certainly no evidence that regular vaginal examinations during labour improve the outcome. We believe that whether in or out of water, interference with the mother's privacy should be kept to a minimum. Examinations should only be performed when they are indicated clinically. Listening to the baby's heart is perfectly possible in the water using a specially adapted doppler machine (sonicaid). If an examination is clinically indicated, then the mother can always get out of the pool.

Many of our mothers have now used our birthing pool. Some have used it for pain relief during the first stage, and have given birth outside the pool. Many have given birth in the pool. They tell us that the experience was good. Few have needed any other form of pain relief. Even the small number of mothers who have had to be transferred to consultant care because of some complication developing in labour, tell us that they valued being in the pool for the time they used it, and that it provided them with adequate pain relief during that time.

In theory, the birth itself should be less traumatic to mother and baby because of the support given by the water to the perineum. Our experience is that women using the pool to give birth have less risk of perineal tears. There is, as yet, no published evidence of which we are aware to confirm this. We certainly would not do episiotomies in the pool unless in some dire emergency.

When the baby is born in the pool, either the midwife lifts it to the surface and the mother can then take her baby, or the baby can be allowed to float to the surface on its own. The baby has been living in water for nine months and will make no attempt to breathe until it emerges into the air, so there is no danger of the baby inhaling the water and drowning in the pool.

The disadvantages of the birthing pool are:

The birthing pool is a relatively new idea and experience with it, although growing, is still at an early stage in most hospitals and community midwifery units.

Michel Odent, one of the pioneers of water birth, says that women in labour are 'attracted to the water.' This is probably true, but some women are certainly not. For them, the idea is unpleasant and would not be a comfortable environment.

Availability of pools is very variable throughout the United Kingdom. Many hospitals have now acquired pools as a result of pressure from women, so the NHS does provide the facility. Unfortunately, not all hospitals have pools, and the rules about who can use them vary between hospitals. Pools are available for hire for use at home, but this can be quite expensive since it is necessary to have the pool in the home for some three to four weeks to be sure of having it available when labour starts.

In hospital, there are often rules about who can use the pool and how it may be used. Some hospitals will not allow women to give birth in the pool and reserve it only for the first stage. Some will not allow the use of any other form of pain relief in the pool, some allow gas and air only. There is some evidence, but this is unconfirmed, that using the birthing pool may slow labour down if the mother enters the pool at an early stage of labour, so some hospitals will not allow women to get into the pool until they have reached five centimetres dilatation of the cervix.

BIRTHING POOL – WHEN TO GET IN?

Opinion We believe that the mother's instinct will usually be right. If she feels it is the right time to get into the pool, then that will probably be right for her whatever the stage of cervical dilatation.

Teresa, at the age of 40, decided that she wanted very much to have her second child born in the birthing pool. She had read about water birth and seen a television programme. She felt strongly that this would be the most relaxing and best environment for her. Her first baby, Tammy, was now 16 and many would have considered Teresa a 'high-risk' case.

We discussed all this with her and she remained very definite about her wishes. The pregnancy was uneventful and Teresa went into labour one Saturday afternoon in our GP unit. By evening, the pool was full and she was walking up and down the ward and occasionally getting into the pool for rest and relaxation. This pattern continued throughout the night and it was not until early on Sunday morning that Teresa stayed in the pool. Joshua was born at about lunchtime on Sunday to the accompaniment of Teresa's favourite country music. The music was turned up louder as the second stage progressed as Teresa seemed to find this helpful. Tammy and Teresa's husband, Colin, were with her throughout labour and at the birth. Teresa was very relaxed throughout a long labour and there was no damage to her perineum, so she required no stitches. She needed no pain relief.

Sandra, like Teresa, had read about water birth and seen TV programmes and felt that this was for her. She was in her early twenties and this was her first pregnancy. Throughout the early part of labour, Sandra was comfortable in the pool and needed no other pain relief; however, in the later part of the first stage, it was clear that progress had ceased and she was becoming exhausted. She was transferred to consultant care and with the aid of augmentation with a syntocinon drip (see later), she delivered two hours later. She said afterwards that she was glad she had been in the pool for most of her labour as she felt relaxed and comfortable for that time.

Michel Odent says that a water birth should not be planned. By this, he means that the water should be used for relaxation and pain relief during labour. If the mother then wishes to stay in the pool to give birth, all well and good, but if she gets out and gives birth on 'dry land', then nothing is lost.

How to get Access to a Birthing Pool or a Water birth

◆ First, ask your Community Midwife or GP. They should know about availability in the local hospital and about hospital policy.

- If they don't have this information, ring your local hospital's director of Midwifery Services.
- If there are no pools available locally, you may have to consider hiring one from a commercial source. Telephone numbers and addresses can often be found in magazines about pregnancy. The Active Birth Centre (see **Addresses**) has pools available for hire.
- If you are going to hire a pool, you will need midwives with experience in water birth to help you use it. Contact your local director of Midwifery Services.
- If you still draw a blank, the only remaining solution is to pay for private midwifery care from an independent midwife. (The Independent Midwives Association will provide a list of local names and contacts.)

The end of the first stage – 'Transition'

'Transition' is used to describe a phase of labour which would not be recognised by most doctors because there is no corresponding anatomical or physiological change to identify it. That certainly doesn't mean that it has no reality. Some midwives and birth teachers describe the time at the end of the first stage of labour as 'Transition'. It is the period when the cervix is almost fully dilated. The contractions are often intense and frequent and it can be a time of considerable psychological and emotional stress or distress. Many women experience fear at this time and we often hear them saying that they are ready to give up, to have a Caesarean section, anything in fact to get away from the situation and the discomfort that they find themselves in.

Michel Odent describes this fear as a positive sign which, he says, may release hormones which stimulate the 'fetal let-down response'. In other words, the fear itself contributes to the quick delivery of the baby. This phase usually lasts only 10 to 20 minutes, and there is little that a mother can do to control what is happening, so it is important that her attendants and supporters are aware of her vulnerability and respond sensitively with gentle, quiet, confident reassurance and encouragement.

We think mothers should be allowed to express their feelings and fears, even by shouting or screaming if they wish to, during this short time. Their attendants should not be too authoritative and should not shout at them unless there are very exceptional circumstances. They should be allowed to follow their instincts, especially with regard to position. Often an 'all-fours' position is the most comfortable at this stage. Changes of position may help, and mothers often feel very restless and want to change position frequently. Sometimes there is an urge to push when the cervix is not quite fully dilated, and this can be confusing and distressing. The knee chest position can be helpful in this case, or if there is an 'anterior lip' of cervix preventing full dilatation. The urge to push is reduced, but the descent of the baby's head and dilatation of the cervix is eased in this position.

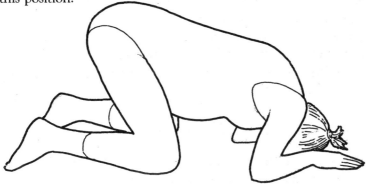

Knee chest position.

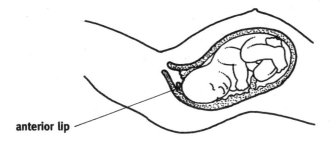

anterior lip

Anterior lip preventing full dilatation.

The Second Stage

When the cervix becomes fully dilated, the baby's head can pass through it into the birth canal. The second stage of labour starts with full dilatation, and ends as the baby's head reaches the perineum and the baby is born. This usually takes no more than an hour, but two hours would be the maximum and a few minutes the minimum. There are often signs that the second stage of labour is happening, which birth attendants can notice, without the need for a vaginal examination. The mother usually feels a strong urge to push or bear down as though she wants to go to the toilet to open her bowels. Indeed, sometimes, as the baby's head descends through the birth canal, there may be some passing of motion which is described as the 'toothpaste sign' because it is like squeezing a tube of toothpaste. Mothers may find this distressing, but their attendants will have seen it all before!

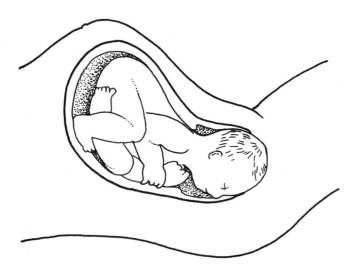

The baby's head beginning to descend through the birth canal.

With the strong contractions of the uterus and the mother's efforts in pushing, the baby descends through the birth canal until the head rests on the perineum. There can then be a feeling of burning tearing in the pelvic floor, 'as if everything were tearing apart', but this is relieved as the head is 'crowned'. The top or crown of the baby's head emerges through the vulva and the shoulders and body follow. Now is the wonderful moment of birth, which though we have seen it hundreds of times, never fails to affect us emotionally. All the pain seems to be forgotten in an instant and replaced by overwhelming joy. Mother and father laugh and cry and so, often, do we.

We like the mother to take the baby straight away, to hold, cuddle, love, perhaps even to feed. We can deal with the tidying up later.

Pushing

It has been practice for many years, for midwives and doctors to encourage, direct or even bully women into pushing, using their abdominal muscles, in the second stage. It is our observation that whatever birth attendants say, do or shout, women will push, or not push, depending on their instincts and ability to do so.

PUSHING

Evidence Research shows conclusively that it is not helpful for the attendants to 'direct' pushing in this way. In fact, the best results come from mothers following their own instincts. Only rarely have we found it necessary to 'take charge' of a mother in the second stage and give her instructions to push.

Nevertheless, established practices in medicine and midwifery are hard to change. If you find yourself in the charge of an attendant who is directing pushing in the old-fashioned way, it may be difficult to protest when in the second stage of labour, in pain and concentrating on other things. Nor may it be appropriate or possible to ask for a change of attendant at this stage. Your partner can come into his own here, and politely ask the attendant to desist (unless you are one of the few who actually finds it helpful).

Positions for the Second Stage and Birth

Common sense tells us that an upright position must help the birth of the baby to be quicker and easier. Further, there is research evidence to support what our common sense tells us. The worst possible position is lying flat on your back on a bed: the baby has to travel uphill in this position (see page 141). Almost any other position is better. The best for each mother will be the one in which she feels most comfortable and which her instincts tell her to get into. She will need support to help her remain upright and to balance the downward forces of the contracting uterus. This support may be given by a partner holding the mother under her arms, or by the use of furniture. (See page 111 and overleaf.)

Supported Squatting

This is the most logical position for the second stage because gravity assists the action of the uterus and the pelvis is as wide open as possible to allow the passage of the baby's head. The sacrum and coccyx are free to move in this position, again making the birth of the head easier. The coccyx will move out of the way during a birth in the squatting position, whereas this movement is restricted in a sitting position. To squat, you need the help of a partner, holding you underneath your arms. He should stand with feet apart and back straight so as not to strain his own back. The mother's weight can rest on her partner's pelvis. He can use anything solid in the room for support, such as a wall, bed or chair. An alternative is for the partner to sit on a chair, supporting the mother between his knees. If your partner has back problems, this can be the best way to protect him.

Supported squatting in this way also has the advantage of freedom to move, even to walk about between contractions if this feels right. The mother should relax into the position, so you need to trust your supporter. Practice before labour starts will make this easier.

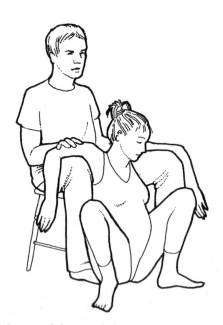

Partner sitting on chair to support mother.

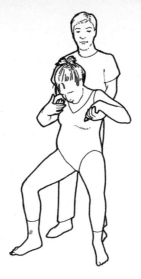

Partner standing behind the mother to give her support while squatting.

All Fours or Kneeling

This is an equally good position, kneeling, with knees well apart, and leaning forward on hands or arms or on cushions, or even beside the bed. It is a particularly useful position if labour is likely to be fast and gives the mother more control. The baby can be passed under the mother's tummy and handed to her as she sits up, or given to her as she rolls over after the birth. This position is helpful if the baby is in the posterior position (looking up as the head is born).

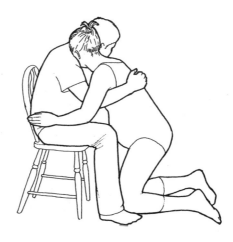

The kneeling position.

Lying on the Side

Although this position does not have the advantage of the help of gravity like the two positions described above, it does still allow the sacrum and coccyx free movement and is certainly better than lying on the back. Some women find this a comfortable position and want to curl up in a ball to give birth.

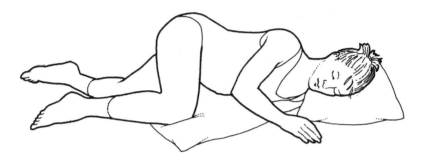

The Perineum – Tears and Episiotomies – To cut or not to cut

We find from experience with women in labour, that the baby's head, if allowed to descend naturally, steadily onto the perineum, will stretch the muscles, ligaments and skin, and allow the delivery of the head without tearing or with minimal tearing in most cases. This seems to us common sense. Our results over a six-year period show that this policy works for our mothers, as our perineal tear rate and episiotomy rates are well below those of the rest of our district.

PERINEUM 'PROTECTION'

Many midwives indulge in the practice of 'protecting' the perineum with a hand or a swab held in the hand as the head is born.

Evidence This procedure is no use in protecting the perineum.

Opinion Many women find it irritating and we feel that it is an unnecessary interference. As we have mentioned before, health professionals find it much more difficult to watch and wait than to do something.

Episiotomy is cutting the perineum when the baby's head descends. The purpose of the cut is to make the delivery easier. The cut may be made either diagonally from the back end of the vulva, or it could be made in the mid-line.

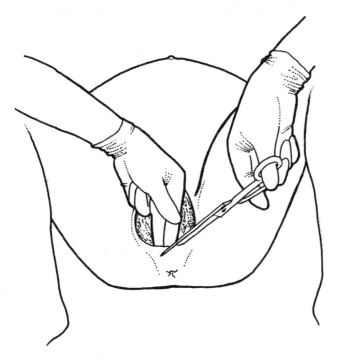

Direction of the cut in an episiotomy.

We feel that episiotomy should only be used when necessary, either to allow the baby to deliver quickly if there are signs of fetal distress, or to allow a forceps delivery. Most hospitals in the UK now have a policy of restricted use of episiotomy.

EPISIOTOMY

Evidence There is no difference in the outcome for mother or baby when policies of liberal use of episiotomy or restricted use of episiotomy are in force. The natural conclusion from the research evidence is that it must be better not to do an episiotomy unless it is absolutely necessary.

The Baby

We feel it is important, unless there are pressing medical reasons, that the baby is given straight away to his or her mother. Babies' immediate needs are for warmth and love. Food may also be given by breast feeding immediately after the birth. Our observation is that some babies seem to want this straight away and others would rather wait a little. Suckling provides a powerful stimulus for separation and delivery of the placenta or afterbirth, but don't be disappointed if your baby doesn't 'catch on' to the idea of feeding immediately. Enough of the hormone oxytocin is released to help with the delivery of the afterbirth simply by the feel of the baby near to the breast.

Babies lose heat quickly, but cuddled up to the mother's body, and wrapped in a towel, your baby will get all the warmth it needs. Physical contact between mother and baby, and also with the father, is really important. You are all going to have to learn to love each other, and the learning starts straight away. It is known that separation of mothers and babies in the early minutes after birth makes 'bonding' or learning to love each other more difficult. Sometimes separation is necessary if the baby or mother have medical problems, but we believe that any separation should be for the least possible time, and this is the policy of most maternity hospitals now.

The baby will probably be a little slippery at first, covered with amniotic fluid and a greasy, creamy substance called vernix which is perfectly normal and natural. He or she may look pink or slightly blue or grey, but the colour rapidly changes to pink as the baby breathes. Some babies cry when they are born, others do not. The cry is not necessary and if the baby is breathing and healthy there is no need for midwives or doctors to slap or pinch them to make them cry, though this is another practice that seems to persist, despite the evidence.

Resuscitation of a Baby

If the baby develops some problem at birth, such as difficulty with breathing, then resuscitation procedures may need to be carried out. Midwives are trained in these procedures but they will usually call the paediatric team in hospital. Sometimes all that is required is the removal of some mucus obstructing the air passages, by use of a suction tube. If it is not possible to solve the problem with the baby in the mother's arms, then the midwife will take the baby and put it on a resuscitation bed. The baby will be placed in a head down position. Breathing will be stimulated or, if necessary, oxygen given through a mask or a tube in the baby's mouth. If Pethidine is the cause of slowness to breathe, the antidote, Naloxone, is given by injection. The baby will be given back to the mother as soon as it is safe.

The Third Stage – Delivery of the Placenta or Afterbirth

After the excitement of the birth of the baby, the mother and her attendants have a rather dull job to do. The placenta or afterbirth, which has for so long been the connection between mother and baby, must be delivered. The uterus will continue to contract after the birth, and as it does so, the placenta separates from the wall of the uterus and is expelled by contractions. Putting the baby to the breast helps to stimulate this process by the release of a hormone called oxytocin. There are two possible approaches to the third stage – the 'expectant' or 'physiological' approach which essentially means just waiting for it to happen naturally, or the '*active*' approach in which things are done to stimulate the process and make it quicker.

The Physiological Third Stage

Waiting and doing nothing are not activities that come naturally to health workers. But to have a physiological third stage these are the two activities that are required most. The placenta will deliver itself if left alone and the only encouragement needed is some suckling by the baby at the breast. The cord need not be cut until the placenta has separated or is delivered. An experienced midwife will know from observing the mother's uterus contracting, and when the placenta has separated, all she needs to do then is to remove it from the vagina. It takes perhaps 15 or 20 minutes, sometimes even up to half an hour. The advantages of a physiological third stage are that no injections are given, there is a smaller risk of retained placenta (the placenta getting stuck and needing to be removed manually under anaesthetic) and probably less pain and discomfort. The disadvantages are the longer wait until everything is finished and the apparent increased risk of post-partum haemorrhage (heavy bleeding) – but we'll discuss this further.

The Active Third Stage

The third stage is considerably speeded up by active management. This consists of birth attendants performing various procedures to hasten the delivery of the placenta. These are: the administration of oxytocin by injection, cutting the cord early, and controlled cord traction which is done by placing a hand on the mother's abdomen to support the uterus, while pulling steadily on the cut end of the umbilical cord. The advantages of this active management are that it gets it all over more quickly.

OXYTOCIN

Evidence There is, without doubt, a substantially lower risk of post-partum haemorrhage associated with the use of oxytocin by means of injection.

However, the disadvantages are that the procedure tends to be more uncomfortable, more interference is required and there is a greater risk of retained placenta. This means that the uterus clamps down on the placenta and prevents it from delivering at all. An anaesthetic is needed to perform a manual removal of the placenta from the uterus. There is also a small risk of side effects from the injection of oxytocin which has very occasionally been associated with fits and cardiac failure in the mother and, rarely, a maternal death. Some hospitals have taken steps to reduce this risk by only using the synthetic hormone syntocinon as an oxytocic in the third stage, and this is certainly the safest policy.

ACTIVE OR PHYSIOLOGICAL?

Evidence about post-partum haemorrhage, although very convincing on the side of using oxytocin, all comes from research in centres where active management of the third stage was normal practice. Nor does it take account of the other elements of active management – cord cutting and controlled cord traction.

Opinion We think that research is needed to compare genuine physiological third stage management, by midwives and doctors experienced in this method, with the use of oxytocin. There is some evidence about when to cut the cord which suggests that it is better for the baby if attendants wait until there are signs of placental separation before cutting.

Induction and Acceleration of Labour

Why?

Induction of labour – 'starting you off' – may be done for reasons related to either the baby's health or the mother's health or both, or occasionally, it must be said, for the convenience of the mother or her attendants. We feel that induction should never be done for the convenience of attendants, but we know it still happens. Valid reasons related to the baby are if there are signs of failure to grow properly (Intra Uterine Growth Retardation or IUGR) or signs of fetal distress – which for the mother may be noticed by reduced fetal movements in the late stages of pregnancy. For the mother, medical problems, especially pre-eclampsia, may be a reason for induction of labour.

How?

Labour can be started by artificial rupture of the membranes (ARM). First a vaginal examination is made. If the cervix is open sufficiently, a plastic hook rather like a crochet hook is passed through the cervix, and the membranes are caught by the hook, which is then withdrawn. The membranes having been broken, there is usually then a rush of fluid from the cervix. Sometimes an ARM is all that is needed to start labour – this might be the case if the pregnancy was close to full term, or past full term and the cervix was already beginning to dilate.

Most commonly though, contractions are stimulated by the administration of oxytocin, a hormone which naturally stimulates contractions when labour starts. This hormone is given through a drip into a vein in the mother's arm. The amount of hormone given is usually controlled, preferably by a mechanical pump which gradually increases the amount of hormone given as labour progresses. The oxytocin is usually a synthetic product called syntocinon. The administration of syntocinon is called 'augmentation of labour'. Syntocinon may also be used to augment labour if it is progressing slowly and there is a need to 'speed things up'.

If the cervix is not sufficiently open to allow passage of the amnihook, then labour may be induced by means of a 'Prostin pessary'. This is a tablet containing a hormone called prostaglandin, which is inserted into the vagina, as close to the cervix as possible. The prostaglandin stimulates dilatation of the cervix and either initiates labour or creates sufficient dilatation of the cervix to allow an ARM to be done.

A similar result can be achieved by having sex because semen contains the same hormone, prostaglandin. Sometimes when a baby is overdue and the mother is being threatened with induction, the advice to have gentle sex will produce a good result.

Forceps Delivery

Why?

A decision to use forceps to deliver the baby is a matter of judgement by the professionals looking after the birth. In the UK, forceps deliveries are usually performed by doctors. There are two main reasons for the decision to use forceps: delay in the second stage and signs of fetal distress. We repeat, there are no hard and fast rules about these indications and the decision depends on the judgement of professionals. **The reasons for the decision and the procedures involved should be explained fully to the mother**. A mother in the second stage of labour is often tired and distressed, so her partner needs to be ready to understand the explanation and to support the mother.

How?

The forceps are put on the baby's head and the doctor pulls with the contractions. The baby's body follows, and is born in the same way as in a 'normal delivery'.

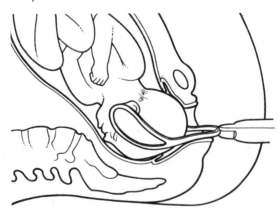

Forceps being used to deliver the baby.

Results

Forceps have the disadvantages of causing damage to the mother's perineum and trauma to the baby's head, though this is usually only temporary. An episiotomy is always necessary. The worst result for the mother can be a 'third-degree tear', which involves the muscles surrounding the anus. This requires an operation to repair it urgently because the result can be incontinence. Because of these disadvantages, it is recommended practice that forceps should not be used, particularly for delay in the second stage, if alternatives are possible. Two alternative procedures are the administration of oxytocin to increase the strength of the contractions, and the use of the ventouse or vacuum extractor.

The Ventouse

The Ventouse consists of a cup which can be metal or plastic, attached to a suction device. The cup is placed on the baby's head and a vacuum produced by suction so that the cup is firmly fixed to the head. The operator can then pull with the contractions to help the birth. The baby develops a swelling of the skin over its head under the cup; this looks a little odd but disappears quickly during the first few days after birth. An episiotomy is not always necessary and there is much less risk of a tear to the mother's perineum with the ventouse than with forceps. The ventouse is usually used by doctors but increasingly midwives are training with it and can use it safely and appropriately.

THE VENTOUSE

Evidence The evidence is that the ventouse is a better, safer instrument than forceps, causing less damage to the mother as long as it is used by an experienced operator, or by juniors under supervision. However, research shows that failure to deliver the baby is more common with the ventouse than with forceps. If failure occurs, then either the forceps can be used or a caesarean section may be necessary.

Gill had a ventouse delivery for Natalie because there was a large amount of meconium present when the membranes ruptured. Gill thought it was fine, but her husband, Mark, was horrified: 'I thought it was horrendous, something out of the mediaeval age.' Gill says, 'They showed me the contraption but I didn't take much in. I didn't feel anything. I dilated very quickly at the end. They said, "Have you got the urge to push?" I said, 'No.'

Trish told me how to push. I got quite annoyed afterwards with the registrar because Trish said, "Just one more push and the baby will come out," but he said, "If she does it right." I didn't like that.' Natalie was fine after some resuscitation, and Gill feels that the experience was quite tolerable and wants to be pregnant again.

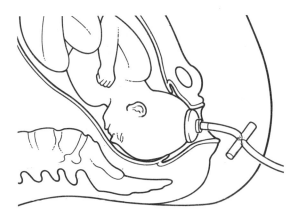

The ventouse used to assist delivery.

Breech Birth

A breech baby is one presenting its bottom, a foot or both feet first to the birth canal. *There is no doubt that this position is more dangerous for the baby.*

BREECH BIRTH

Evidence Breech babies are more at risk than those presenting their heads first. What is unclear is whether this higher risk relates to delivery by the breech or to some other factor affecting breech babies. Because of the known risks, there is an increasing tendency to deliver breech babies by caesarean section. There is no evidence either way at present as to whether this is a good policy or not.

To put the situation very simply, perhaps over-simply, breech birth by the vaginal route carries a higher risk for the baby, caesarean section carries a higher risk for the mother. Research is needed to resolve this question.

It is advisable for breech babies to be born in hospital and in a Consultant unit because of the greater risk to the baby. Specifically, there is a risk of damage to the baby's head and brain as the head follows last through the pelvis. This is particularly true for premature births, and the breech presentation is more common in premature births. Another risk is that of disproportion – the pelvis is not big enough for the head to be born – but this is becoming less common as women become healthier due to improved standards of living.

If your baby presents as a breech when you go into labour, your chance of having a caesarean is now very considerable. If all is well and you are able to have a vaginal birth, then common sense would suggest that the principles of anatomy and physiology still apply, and the best position for delivery would be a supported squat from a standing position. Few midwives or obstetricians, however, have experience of this position and may feel uncomfortable unless the mother is lying on the delivery bed.

Caesarean Section

Why?
This operation may be done for the benefit of the baby or of the mother, or both. Most commonly nowadays, it is done for reasons to do with the health of the baby and the most common reason given is that the baby is showing signs of fetal distress during the first stage of labour. A caesarean might be indicated for the baby's benefit before labour starts if there are signs of placental insufficiency – the baby is not growing adequately or receiving adequate nutrition. Problems for the mother that affect the baby may indicate the need for a caesarean. Pelvic disproportion is less common now than in the first half of the century. This means that the mother's pelvis is too small to allow the passage of the baby's head.

Increasingly, caesareans are performed for breech presentation and may be necessary for brow or shoulder presentations. Antepartum haemorrhage may mean a caesarean is urgently necessary, potentially to save two lives. Severe pre-eclampsia may also be an indication for caesarean section. Failure of the uterus to contract properly in labour is another indication of this.

There has been a rapid increase in the number of caesareans performed in the western world during the last ten years. In Britain, the present rate is about 20% and rising. There does not seem to be a genuine medical or obstetric reason for this increase and there is certainly no evidence that this increase has been associated with an improvement in perinatal mortality, maternal mortality or the health of mothers and babies. The World Health Organisation has become concerned about this trend and has stated standards for rates of caesarean section which its experts think are reasonable for most hospitals in western countries. WHO recommends a rate of 10% or less in an ordinary district general hospital and 15% in special centres in which more difficult cases are dealt with. Arithmetic shows, if these standards were followed, that in an average local hospital with a caesarean section rate of 20% and 2,000 births per year, 200 women had unnecessary caesareans in one year.

In our practice, the caesarean section rate has remained at approximately seven and a half per cent for the last six years despite an increase from 11% to 22% in the local health district. We think we have helped our mothers to avoid caesareans by giving them information, although there may well be other factors involved. One of the most common complaints that mothers make about caesareans is that they were not given enough information about the operation beforehand. We recognise that many caesareans are done in an emergency situation and it is not possible or appropriate to spend time explaining the pros and cons of the procedure. We feel that mothers should have this information ready before they go into labour and so we discuss caesareans fully in our antenatal sessions.

How?

Most caesareans are done by a making a cut in the skin just above the pubic bones, in the 'bikini line'. The bladder is kept out of the way with a retractor, which an assistant usually holds. A cut is made in the peritoneum, the thin membrane which lines the abdominal cavity. A small cut is made in the lower part of the uterus, and the operator then inserts fingers to widen the hole. The surgeon then puts a hand in the uterus to lift the baby's head out while an assistant presses on the top of the uterus to push the baby out. Sometimes forceps are used to lift out the head. Ergometrine is given by injection, which encourages the uterus to contract. The placenta is then delivered. The baby, meanwhile, can be resuscitated, if necessary, or given to the mother if the operation is performed under epidural or spinal block. The surgeon must then sew everything back together carefully and this usually takes quite a bit longer than the delivery of the baby.

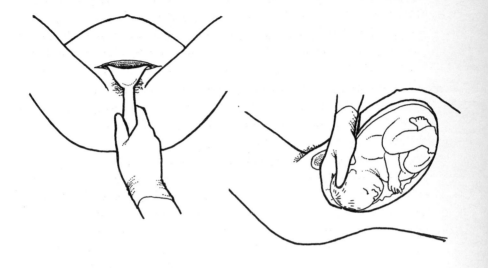

The womb being opened with a retractor after the initial incision.   **The surgeon lifting the baby's head.**

Anaesthetics

The operation can be done in the same way as major operations of other kinds, under general anaesthetic, in which case the mother is not conscious during the procedure. It is more common now to use epidural or spinal anaesthesia to do the operation. This is safer for the mother and has the great benefit to her that she is awake during the birth and can see and hold the baby straight away as long as there are no problems. In most cases and hospitals, fathers can be present in the operating theatre. The epidural or spinal block is given in the same way as we described earlier, or if the operation is done when there is already an epidural in, then it merely needs topping up before the operation starts. Mothers who have experienced this say that they feel nothing except the sensation of someone rummaging around inside their stomachs – which is strange, but tolerable. Many experience some fear, before the operation begins, that they will feel pain. Before the operation, some shaving of abdominal or pubic hair may be needed. A catheter is inserted into the bladder to empty it. A screen is put up between the mother's chest and abdomen so that she can't see what is going on. Most mothers like this!

Complications

Reading about the complications of any kind of operation can be somewhat alarming for someone planning to have that operation. Many operations are performed every day in hospitals throughout the country. Disasters, thankfully, are rare because of the skill of the surgeons, anaesthetists, midwives and technicians who are involved in the care of patients. Nevertheless, despite everybody's best efforts, all surgery carries some risk for the patient. We find that discussing the risks openly with our mothers helps them to understand this and to prepare for complications which we all hope won't occur.

Caesarean section is a major operation. The complications are the same as for all major surgery with the addition of some things that are specific to caesarean section. As with any other major operation, there is a very small risk of death during a caesarean section. Haemorrhage is probably the most serious and life-threatening complication. Surgeons doing caesarean sections pay particular attention to this because the angles of the incision in the uterus may tear as the baby's head is being delivered, and there are large arteries close by. It is part of the surgeon's skill and training to prevent excessive bleeding. In very severe cases of haemorrhage it may be necessary to do a hysterectomy to stop the bleeding.

Pulmonary Embolism (PE)

This is a blood clot which settles in the lungs. It is an uncommon, but serious complication of all major operations, and is the most common cause of death associated with caesarean section. Surgeons and midwives are keen to identify patients who are at risk of PE and to try to prevent it. People at risk are those who have a previous history of clotting problems such as deep vein thrombosis or thrombophlebitis, people who are very overweight, and heavy smokers. Getting mobile as soon as possible after the operation reduces the risk. Physiotherapists usually impress on patients the need to do leg exercises after the operation.

Infection

This is a common complication of all surgery. Because of the emergency nature of caesarean section, infection is perhaps more likely than for other operations. To prevent this, many surgeons give antibiotics before the operation whenever possible.

Wound dehiscence

This means that the wound opens up again after the operation. It is more likely with caesarean section than with other abdominal operations because the bowel often becomes distended with gases during the first few days after the operation and the abdominal muscles tend to be lax.

After the Op

Our mothers tell us it can take from six months to a year to recover fully from the operation. Most surgeons tell their patients that it takes three months to recover from most major operations. People vary enormously in their powers of healing and recovery.

In the immediate post-operative period, in hospital, mothers are usually encouraged to be up and walking about the next day. This reduces the risk of late complications including pulmonary embolism. They are encouraged to do exercises, especially of the legs and feet, again to prevent the problem of embolism. There is post-operative pain in the abdomen and in the wound area. Most mothers are given strong analgesics (pain killers) such as morphine for the first 24 hours, and less potent ones such as paracetamol after that. Mothers are encouraged (some would say made) to look after their babies completely themselves from the beginning. They tell us it can be quite hard doing this when somewhat groggy from the effects of anaesthesia and morphine, and still experiencing pain, but most are glad they did it. The usual stay in hospital is now four days after the operation if there are no complications. Coming home can be a bit of a shock because much is expected of mothers, especially if there are children at home already. Families need to be sympathetic and to allow mothers some time for recovery from a major operation.

Amanda's story – two very necessary caesareans

At about 30 weeks into her first pregnancy, Amanda's blood pressure went up to 150/100. She had protein in her urine and considerable fluid retention (oedema). She was referred to the hospital antenatal clinic, from where she was admitted to the ward. After two weeks in hospital, the decision was taken that because her blood pressure was continuing to rise and she was becoming more ill, the baby should be delivered by caesarean section. (Not even the most strident critic of obstetric intervention could find fault with this decision, we think.) Amanda had her first caesarean under general anaesthetic.

Although everyone accepts that her operation was necessary and possibly life-saving for her and her baby, Robert, Amanda still feels that she did not have enough information about the operation and its consequences beforehand. She feels that because Robert was born while she was under general anaesthesia, she did not know him very well at first and it took longer to get to know and love him than her second child, Bethany, who was also born by caesarean, but this time with epidural anaesthesia. She held Bethany immediately after she was born. Bethany was born two years after Robert, and again Amanda's blood pressure went up at 30 weeks. After both operations, Amanda says that the third day was the worst; the wind in her tummy was bad at that stage, the wound and stitches were most painful, and she felt at her lowest. She says that peppermint worked very well to relieve the wind. When out of hospital she felt very tired, but fortunately her husband took time off work and did everything at home except feed the babies, as Amanda wished to breast feed. She feels that it took about a year to recover from the operation in each case.

A story of two perhaps avoidable caesareans

The authors personally witnessed the events of this story. We feel that the people involved should remain anonymous. We'll call the mother Diane. Her first pregnancy was normal and she went into labour at full term. She was admitted to the GP unit at her local hospital. Her doctor and midwife were both in attendance. Labour proceeded slowly, as is often the case with first pregnancies. Diane became very tired after about ten hours in labour, and quite distressed. She had not progressed very far – the cervix was still at about four centimetres. We decided to transfer her to the consultant unit for assessment and probably for augmentation of labour with syntocinon. Diane did not like being moved or disturbed during her labour. Many mothers have this feeling of wanting to curl up and to be left alone.

In the labour ward a midwife came to Diane. She explained that Diane would be able to adopt whatever position she liked and that she would be well looked after.

However, 20 minutes later, she wanted to listen to the fetal heart and asked Diane to roll over onto her back. Diane did not want to do this. She was instructed in no uncertain terms that she must comply! From then on everything seemed to deteriorate. Diane became more and more distressed and less 'co-operative'. Eventually a junior doctor (a registrar) was called. He perhaps unwisely wrote in the case notes 'patient refuses examination – for caesarean section'. It seemed to Diane and to us that this was something that had been inflicted as a punishment.

Diane's second pregnancy resulted in a late miscarriage, two years later. Following this she became pregnant again. This time she had consultant care throughout and bravely took part in some research about the treatment of late miscarriage. She had her second baby by caesarean section under spinal anaesthetic. We can't help asking ourselves, if her first birth been handled more sensitively, would she have needed the first caesarean, and therefore the second?

Why are Caesarean Sections becoming more common?

The factors involved in caesarean sections are many and complex. There are two undisputed facts:

1. There has been no apparent change in the medical or physical condition of women or their babies in the last ten years that would explain a doubling of the caesarean section rate.
2. Neither has this increase in caesareans been shown to have improved the outcome for mother or baby in terms of perinatal mortality or maternal mortality, or morbidity (diseases and complications).

We believe that obstetric specialists, in this country at least, act with the best of intentions, and genuinely believe that decisions they make are in the best interests of the mothers they care for. They work hard, often under pressure, and with diminishing resources afforded by the NHS. They are subjected to increasing litigation against them when things go wrong.

Fear of litigation among obstetricians is probably one factor in the increasing caesarean rate, indeed some obstetricians admit this. With families of their own to support, and a rewarding career at stake, who can blame them? Obstetricians also tell us that increasingly they are put under pressure by a small but growing number of women who actually ask for or demand caesarean section.

Increasing use of technology such as intra-partum fetal monitoring has been shown to be responsible for some of the increase in operative deliveries.

WHAT HAPPENS WHEN THINGS GO WRONG?

....

Sue's Story

Sue had a very difficult year. She had one daughter aged 15 by her first husband who had recently died. Having re-married, she was delighted to be pregnant. Aged 35, having had no problems with pregnancy or labour in her first pregnancy, she opted for care by her family doctor and midwife and delivery in our local GP unit. She was one of our most regular attenders at the clinic, contributing to the discussion and endearing herself to the whole group because of her sense of humour.

Sue appeared 'larger for dates' from the early stages, but ultrasound scans showed that the baby was normal, there was only one baby present and the liquor surrounding the baby was also normal. She reached the end of her pregnancy with no problems except that it was obvious that the baby was going to be a big one.

Sue went into labour one afternoon, a week after her expected date. She went to the GP unit where an experienced midwife attended her. Just before she went to the hospital her waters broke. When the GP unit midwife examined her, she found that the baby had passed fresh meconium. This is a warning sign, but usually leads to no problems as long as extra care is taken of the baby during labour. The midwife quite correctly transferred Sue to the consultant unit as soon as she discovered this.

Sue's labour continued throughout the night, during which the baby's heart was monitored. There appeared to be no problem. At 7am, Sue entered the second stage of labour. The baby's head was visible and was born. At this point, a tragedy occurred. The baby's shoulders would not come out. The midwife looking after Sue immediately summoned help from the doctor on call, and continued trying to deliver the baby. An episiotomy was made. The doctor arrived and the baby was delivered after six minutes from when the head was born. This should still have given the baby sufficient chance to recover, but unfortunately he died of asphyxia. They called him Matthew. He weighed 10lb and was quite perfect.

No one really understands why Matthew died. Sue had received excellent care in labour and all the right things were done. He was a big baby, but this is usually a sign of health and bigger babies are born quite safely. Sue is not a small person. Even after he got stuck (this is known as shoulder dystocia), it should have been possible to resuscitate him.

Despite all the efforts of midwives and doctors, despite all the advances in medical technology, we still have to face tragedies like Matthew's. In the United Kingdom, as in most advanced nations, perinatal mortality is less than ten per thousand (ten babies die at birth or in the first week of life for every thousand live births). This represents a great improvement over the last 30 years. In 1964, the perinatal mortality rate was between 20 and 30 per thousand. In Third World countries, the perinatal mortality may be as high as 10%.

After the birth, Sue and her husband Dave were encouraged to see Matthew and to hold him. They were given photographs and an appointment with a counsellor, and an opportunity for a funeral service. The mothers in the group were very distressed when they were given the news, but they all said that they were glad we had told them about it. Some of them contacted Sue and she has valued their support.

It was six years since a baby had died in the practice and we also found the experience very distressing. We supported each other and also felt better for open discussion of our feelings with the mothers.

What Happens When Things Go Wrong?

In the event of a tragedy like Sue and Dave's, there should be help and support available in the hospital or the community, both immediately and in the weeks following. The hospital chaplain is on hand to perform services such as baptism, and to offer spiritual support and counselling, and secular counsellors are also available to help with bereavement.

Sue said that the worst thing for her was leaving the hospital. She felt the loss most as she walked out of the building empty-handed.

Information

Most parents want to know, as Dave and Sue did, exactly what went wrong in such a tragic event. Most people don't want to blame anyone or to exact revenge, but if there has been a mistake, the overwhelming feeling most people have is that it must not happen to anyone else.

Matthew's death was discussed by the hospital doctors and midwives at a meeting. The case notes were reviewed thoroughly to see if any lessons could be learnt. The consultant in charge of their case went over the events carefully with Sue and Dave, and they feel satisfied, as all the staff involved were, that everything had been done that was possible to help Matthew. They feel that there has been an honest and open investigation and discussion of their case and this has been a great comfort to them. Misunderstandings in such situations seem to arise because there is seen to be a lack of openness and honesty in investigating the facts and giving information to parents. Hopefully this is now becoming less common and an open approach is the norm.

Help with Grief

We would all like to hope that when tragedy strikes, the support of our family and friends is the most valuable. Professionals who have been involved in the case should also be sympathetic and helpful. All these people will be sharing in the grief and sometimes when grief becomes a dominant feeling and persists in interfering with day to day living, we can benefit from the help of a disinterested counsellor – someone who is sympathetic from outside the situation. There are organisations dedicated to helping in such situations. The addresses are given below:

Compassionate Friends,
53 North Street,
Bristol BS3 1EN
(0117 953 0965)
They have information about local groups for counselling.

Foundation for Study of Infant Deaths
(Cot Death Research and Support),
35 Belgrave Square,
London SW1X 8QB
(24-hour helpline 0171 235 1721)

Stillbirth and Neonatal Death Society (SANDS)
28 Portland Place,
London W1N 4DE
(0171 436 7940; helpline 0171 436 5881)

CHAPTER NINE

NOW WHAT? – THE NEW BABY

....

Preparing for the New Baby

Most (probably all!) of the parents we talk to agree that the coming of their first baby was the biggest change in their lives. Life becomes so different, priorities change so much that many feel nothing could prepare them for this change. Parents who have already had one baby will know what to expect to a certain extent, but even then every baby is different, will behave differently and make different demands. First-time mothers might like to try this exercise: Make a plan of your day on the 24-hour clock face below, dividing the day into sections. How long do you sleep? What time do you spend eating, working, relaxing?

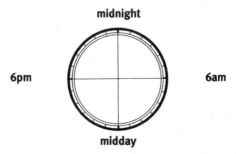

Now do the same, imagining that you have a new baby. How will your day look? How will your sleep be affected? What time will you have for relaxing?

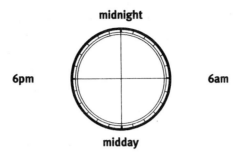

Adjusting to the New Baby

Babies change very rapidly from the moment of birth. Most parents say that the time of babyhood seems very short when they are able to look back on it with their now older or grown-up children. Indeed it is a very short time, for by the end of the first year, babies are ready to walk. After two years, most are saying short sentences and after four years, they are ready to go to school. In the perspective of a life, babyhood is a very brief period. It can be very hard work, but make the most of it! It doesn't last long.

You can enjoy watching the baby grow and develop every day. There is a lot of love to be shared, but this too has to develop. Sometimes there is 'love at first sight' for the mother, but the baby will have to get to know its parents as it becomes more aware of them. Researchers who have studied mothers and their babies find that communication between mother and baby develops very quickly and soon the baby and mother develop eye contact. Newborn babies can certainly see, contrary to some myths, but they seem to be unable to focus on distant objects at first. Perhaps it is not by chance that a baby's optimal focusing point appears to be about the distance between its mother's arm, as she cradles it, and her face. One of the first images a baby perceives, therefore, will be its mother's face, especially her eyes.

This is not just sentimental speculation. These early relationships between mother and baby are known to be important in the child's and adult's later emotional and psychological development. Babies are also able to hear and have got used to sounds within the womb. These sounds will be mainly the sounds of the mother's heart beat, which the newborn baby can hear when it is cuddled up close to the mother's breast. This familiar sound may be comforting. Research shows that babies respond to external sounds such as music while still in the womb. Other senses such as smell, taste and feel are also important to babies. As one expert put it, 'Babies, they're smarter than they look!'

In the first week after birth, practical matters such as feeding, bathing and changing the baby's nappies can become the focus of a mother's life. These things have to be done, but can they be done as part of the growing and developing relationship between mother and baby, and father and baby? How can new mothers and fathers maintain their love for each other and for their new child and for their older children, while at the same time meeting the practical demands of caring for the new baby? Each family will develop its own answers to these questions in its own way. We don't think we can provide the answers, but one thing stands out as a great help to new mothers – **the support of other mothers**.

Our experience is that after the birth and the excitement involved, after the visitors and grandparents have gone home, after father has gone back to work, a new mother can feel very alone and isolated with her baby at home. Am I doing this right? Is this normal? Am I being a good mother?

There is a lot of pressure, both internal and external, to be a 'good mother'. Striving for perfection in mothering can itself be very stressful and daunting. The renowned paediatrician and child psychotherapist, Winnicott, spoke and wrote of 'the good enough mother'. Being ill with stress and worry may jeopardise the ability to be 'good enough'. It may be best for first-time mothers to settle for being 'good enough'. Can you, as a new mother, establish your priorities, which for most will be developing loving relationships in the family. Maybe you can let other less important matters slip in these early crucial weeks of the new baby's life.

We've found that mothers who know other mothers feel more confident and more relaxed about their babies. Another mother who is experiencing the same concerns, fears and joys can be a wonderful help – just a chat on the phone can provide so much reassurance. We find that these relationships between mothers develop in our antenatal clinic groups and continue afterwards. So, to prepare for the new baby, if we could give one piece of advice only, it would be **get to know other mothers**.

Mum Knows Best

In the completely new experience of a baby, mothers can find themselves overwhelmed with advice from both amateurs and professionals. Midwives, doctors, health visitors, broadcasters and writers of books all seem eager to press advice upon them, to say nothing of mothers and grandmothers and neighbours. Sometimes this can be bewildering and there can be conflicting advice. Who should the mother believe? Our own experience is that in all this confusion the best course of action for a mother is to follow her own instincts. They usually won't lead her astray. Thank the people politely for their advice and then **do what you think is best**. To would-be advisers of mothers, including the professionals, we would like to say that what mothers need most is not advice but **support**. Yes, what you are doing is OK. I didn't do it that way, but if it works for you, fine. Yes, I had that experience, I handled it this way, but there could be other ways. Have you thought of doing that? What about trying . . . ?

New mothers may come under pressure, from their own mothers or experienced friends, to establish routines. Failure to fit in with someone else's expectations can be stressful too. Just as in preparing for pregnancy and for birth, new mothers can gather a lot of information and listen to advice, but the objective should be for themselves to make their own choices and decisions. What suits you and your own baby will be best. Every baby is a little individual and this becomes very obvious from early on. What is right for one baby may not be right for another.

The First Week

The baby's needs at first are very simple. **Food, warmth and love**. Babies also need basic hygiene – they need their nappies to be changed and to be kept clean. At first, the new baby spends quite a lot of time asleep, but this is not necessarily at night-time when its parents want to be asleep. At first, mothers (and fathers too) may need to get their own rest when the baby does. Gradually, over the first year of life, routines of bedtime get established. Some babies seem to adapt to the needs of their parents very quickly and sleep through the night from an early stage. Others take much longer to adapt and we have known haggard parents of three-year-old children who are still waking regularly in the night. These are exceptional, but unfortunately there doesn't seem to be any way of predicting how children will sleep or of altering the process.

Babies will cry from the first day and this is good, since crying is the only way of audible communication a new baby has. Mothers soon get to know their baby's cry and respond to it. Crying may mean 'I'm hungry' or 'I'm too cold' or too hot, or 'my nappy needs changing', or just 'I'm here, I want some attention please!' The cry is quite a disturbing sound and a continually crying baby can be very distressing to its parents. Continual crying is quite a common reason for mothers to bring their baby to the doctor. It is very unusual indeed to find a medical reason for crying. Ill babies, in fact, usually cry less than well ones. If you have problems about your baby's crying, we recommend Sheila Kitzinger's excellent book, *The Crying Baby*.

The Midwife

The midwife's role doesn't end when the baby is born. She will visit during the first week of the new baby's life and can help and give support with feeding and all aspects of baby care, as well as with the mother's own health. Mothers tell us that the support of an experienced and motherly midwife is invaluable in reassuring and encouraging a new mother to develop confidence in herself and her own abilities as a mother.

Baby Equipment

Very little is needed for the first week or two of a baby's life. Remembering the needs for food, warmth, love and cleanliness, the basic 'kit' could consist of the following items.

Checklist for Baby Equipment

- Clothes – three or four first-size 'babygrows' and the same number of vests
- Sheets and blankets
- Somewhere to sleep – a 'carry cot', a crib, a pram or even a drawer will suffice
- A bowl for washing – a kitchen bowl will do just as well as a more expensive baby bath
- Some first-size nappies – most people now use disposable nappies and the technology of these has certainly resulted in an easier life for mothers, and probably more comfort for babies. Terry nappies, however, are finding popularity again because they are more environmentally friendly and cost a lot less in the long run. There's the disadvantage of washing, however
- Baby wipes for use when out of the house
- Food – no equipment is needed for breast feeding; two bottles and teats and some sterilising equipment for bottle feeding

The Cord

This needs a little attention in the first week of life, before it drops off. The remnant of the umbilical cord attaching the baby to the placenta, which is cut just after birth, will remain attached to the baby's tummy in the first week. During this week it will shrivel up and fall off, leaving a 'tummy button' or umbilicus. Cleaning with warm water, and the application of some Sterzac powder each time the baby is bathed, is all that's needed. Occasionally the cord can look messy but it's very rare that any treatment other than simple hygiene is needed.

Jaundice

This is normal, especially in breast-fed babies, in whom it can last for up to six weeks. The baby looks an orangey-yellow colour. Ultra-violet light is effective in reducing the level of jaundice. In practice, you can give your baby this 'treatment' by taking him or her out for a walk in the fresh air, or simply by putting the pram by a window. Even in winter, the sun's rays produce enough ultra violet for some therapeutic effect. The jaundice will clear naturally, anyway.

The cause is a yellow pigment called *bilirubin*, which is produced in our blood. The liver usually deals with this pigment but a newborn baby's liver may not be fully developed at first so that the pigment appears in the skin. Normal (physiological) jaundice appears when the baby is about two days old and usually disappears after the first week. There are other causes of jaundice, so if it doesn't disappear you should ask your midwife, health visitor or doctor about it.

Preparing for Twins

Twins create at least twice as much work in feeding, dressing, changing and generally caring for two babies instead of one. Being prepared for this could help. Mothers and fathers will both lose a lot of sleep in the first few months and the demands during the day will also be increased. Two pieces of common sense advice are: get as much help as you can, from family and friends and from the social services department, who may be able to provide 'home help'. Secondly, don't plan to take on anything new at work or in leisure time during the first few months because most of your energies will be needed in child care.

There is a network of local Twin Clubs, which provide mutual support for parents of twins, from other parents of twins. Knowing how someone else has coped or are coping at present can be a great help. Your health visitor or midwife should have the details of these.

FEEDING

Breast is Best

There can be no doubt that breast-feeding is best for both mother and baby. The advantages of breast-feeding are:

- breast milk is the perfect food for baby – it contains all the nourishment that a baby needs;
- breast milk is adaptable – its composition changes as the baby grows, providing the right content at the right time;
- breast milk is easily digested by baby;
- breast milk contains antibodies and nutrients which protect baby from illness;
- breast-fed babies suffer from fewer allergies than bottle-fed babies;
- breast milk is convenient – no need for carrying equipment around when travelling and no bottles to fetch or to make up;
- breast milk is at exactly the right temperature for baby;
- breast-feeding actually helps mothers to regain fitness and figure after the birth;
- breast-feeding is emotionally satisfying for mother and baby – it helps in the process of getting to know each other and sharing love;
- there is evidence that breast-feeding reduces the risk of breast cancer for mothers;
- breast-feeding has no cost.

Every mother has the ability to breast-feed, but it is a skill that needs to be learnt, and it requires determination and practice. Putting the baby to the breast immediately after birth can help to start breast-feeding. This also helps with the separation of the placenta.

Colostrum

For the first two or three days after birth, the breasts produce colostrum which is a yellowy clear fluid. The milk itself begins production by about the third day. Nature has provided in colostrum the perfect food for the newborn baby. It contains antibodies which prevent infection, it has laxative properties which help to clear the baby's bowel of meconium, ready for absorption of the milk, and it contains exactly the right nutrients that a newborn baby needs. Sucking colostrum helps to stimulate production of milk. The newborn baby needs to be close to its mother and allowed to suck as often as it wishes and for as long as it needs. This can be quite demanding, but it is only going to last for a few days and will be worth the effort for both baby and mother.

The First Milk

Two to four days after the birth, the first milk starts to come in. This can be uncomfortable and often coincides with the low point that many women experience between the third and fifth day. Mothers often feel 'weepy' and cry for no apparent reason. The breasts can feel hot and sore (this is known as engorgement). It will last for only 24 to 48 hours. It's important not to give up at this point, tempting though it may seem. Continued sucking actually relieves the engorgement, and if one side is worse than the other, which is often the case, don't be tempted to use the more comfortable side, because this will only make the other one worse. A warm bath may bring some relief, especially if you can lie on your tummy. Good support for the breasts from a nursing bra will be helpful. If they are hot and look red and inflamed, homoeopathic Belladonna 6c taken every two hours has helped many of our mothers. Another trick that they tell us is helpful is to apply warm flannels to the breast before a feed and cold ones afterwards. It's important to tell someone how you feel and receive comfort and support during this time. Husbands or partners need to be especially sympathetic and prepared to take a bit of abuse.

Sore, cracked nipples can be helped by homoeopathic Calendula cream, which will not harm the baby. Homoeopathic Phytolacca taken orally can also help.

The Art of Breast-feeding

A most important point: **every mother should be able to produce enough milk to satisfy her baby**. No one should ever feel that they are not producing enough milk. The milk is produced by a reflex, so the more you feed, the more milk is produced. The baby in fact stimulates exactly what he or she needs by sucking. A newborn baby's stomach is about the size of a golf ball, so it needs feeding frequently with small amounts.

Following from this point, **there is never any need to supplement**

breast-feeding with bottle feeds. The research evidence shows that this is unnecessary and that it acts as a disincentive for both mother and baby. We still come across mothers who have been advised by midwives, doctors or health visitors to give their babies a 'top up'. This seems to go on despite the circulation of policy documents, publication of evidence and training courses. If you get this sort of advice, thank the person politely, and then just continue with your own method! We hope this will be breast-feeding alone.

Many mothers give their babies dummies because the babies enjoy sucking and the dummy gives them comfort and tends to 'keep them quiet'. However, sucking a dummy reduces the time a baby will spend sucking at the breast and therefore this may reduce milk production.

Another principle to understand is that the milk changes its composition throughout a feed. When feeding starts, the milk is more watery and at the end it tends to be thicker and creamier. Because of this, it is better to finish feeding from one side, emptying the breast, before changing over to the other.

The reflex that stimulates the release of milk (the 'let down reflex') may take two minutes from the start of suckling. Sometimes mothers feel a tingling sensation when this is occurring. This is another reason why it is important to start feeding on one side and not to change to the other side until the first side is empty. Unfortunately, we still find that mothers have been advised by professionals to change sides after two minutes which is totally wrong.

'Latching On'

Positioning the baby correctly on the breast will help the baby to feed efficiently and to prevent the nipples from becoming sore.

- ◆ Sit in a comfortable chair with good support for your back. Our osteopath advises mothers to alternate the sides they start feeding from in order to preserve symmetry and not to put too much strain on one side. Feeding can also be done by lying on your side with the baby cuddled up close. After having a caesarean, this may be the most comfortable position.
- ◆ When the baby touches the nipple, a reflex makes it open its mouth wide. It is important to wait for the mouth to open wide.
- ◆ The baby should be facing the breast, and the baby's mouth should be over the whole of the nipple and the surrounding brown area (the areola).

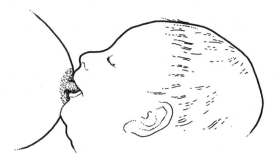

The baby is sucking on the nipple *only*. This does not allow proper suckling and is painful for the mother.

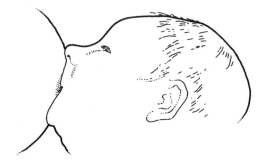

The baby is correctly sucking on the whole nipple and areola. This results in efficient feeding and should be comfortable for the mother.

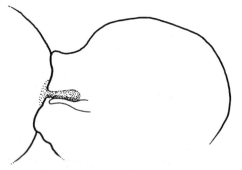

In this correct position the nipple is at the *back* of the baby's throat and he/she can use the tongue for suckling.

- The milk comes from the breast, not the nipple, and the baby's tongue presses the milk from the ducts in the breast through the nipple into its throat. The nipple should be at the back of the baby's throat.
- It is sucking on the nipple which makes for sore nipples and an unsatisfied baby because little or no milk will be produced this way.
- The best way is to feed your baby **on demand**. At first, this may mean feeding almost continually, but very soon the baby will establish his or her own routine. The gaps between feeds will become longer and the feeding time shorter.
- Feed the baby until he or she has had enough, when probably the baby will fall into a happy sleep. Sometimes a baby will suck for comfort after he/she has had enough milk for food. They may slide off the nipple and then give some quivering fluttering sucks. After a few of these it's time to take them off when they should settle down.
- Don't time feeds and don't weigh the baby before and after to check that it has had enough. It certainly has had enough!

Care of Breast-feeding Mothers

Breast-feeding mothers need to take care of themselves and to be taken care of by their husbands, partners, friends and relations. They need:

- A good diet – no particular foods are to be recommended for breastfeeding but a good balanced diet of the sort we described in Chapter One is the best. Be careful with alcohol, smoking, caffeine and drugs (including pharmaceuticals); all of these get into the milk, so you will be feeding them to the baby.
- Rest and relaxation – breastfeeding does take quite a lot of energy, and this needs to be recognised by the mother and her family. At first, when feeding may be frequent, it is beneficial for the mother to rest when the baby is asleep. Breastfeeding, in fact, tends to make the mother rest.
- Emotional support – it can be very draining emotionally to have this small dependent person making frequent and insistent demands on you. Husbands, partners and family need to understand this and to respond sensitively.
- Advice – if problems arise, there are local breastfeeding counsellors available to give advice and support. These are often associated with

the NCT or the La Leche League (see addresses at the end of this chapter). Your local surgery or health clinic may have a breast-feeding counsellor attached. If you can't find someone, ask your midwife, health visitor or doctor. Sadly, our experience is that advice from health professionals on breastfeeding is variable in quality, so for the safest advice, go to the breastfeeding counsellor.

A mother has to find the balance between the baby's needs and her own. She may need to decide when she can afford to indulge the baby completely and when she needs five minutes for a shower or a bath, or to prepare a meal. Babies do not come to harm by being left to cry for brief periods while these necessary things are done.

Expressing Breast Milk

If you want to go out for an evening without the baby, it is perfectly possible to do so without resorting to bottle feeds by expressing some breast milk by hand or with a pump. The milk can be stored in a fridge for 24 hours, or for up to three months in the freezer.

Breast-feeding Checklist

♦ Relax before you start and make sure you're comfortable, with everything you need to hand. Shoulders back, feet supported.
♦ Support your baby behind the shoulders, **never** behind the head as this prevents a good position on the breast.
♦ Position the baby, close to you with his/her chest and tummy touching your chest and tummy. **Chest to chest, chin to breast**.
♦ Line up the baby's nose with your nipple.
♦ Wait for the baby to open his/her mouth, and then wait a little longer until the mouth is wide open.
♦ Bring your baby to the breast by using your hand behind the baby's shoulders. Never try to put the breast into the baby's mouth.
♦ Remember the baby feeds from the breast by pressing with the tongue. The nipple should be at the back of the baby's mouth.
♦ If feeding hurts, take the baby off the breast by sliding your little finger into the corner of the mouth and along the nipple. Try again, taking your time and relaxing.

The baby is feeding well when:

- It doesn't hurt;
- The baby takes long slow sucks;
- The cheeks don't suck in and out with feeding;
- The baby doesn't make clicking noises;
- He/she is on his side and close to you;
- He/she is feeding contentedly.

Bottle-feeding

Some mothers prefer to bottle-feed because they feel that they can cope better this way. Be sure that this is really for you before you give up the advantages of breastfeeding. Bottle-feeding should not be continued after one year because of the risk of dental decay.

Nutrition

Most artificial milks are produced from cows' milk. The protein, fat and salt content of cows' milk is difficult for the newborn baby to digest, so these are reduced to make the milk as close to breast milk as possible. Bottle-fed babies will get enough of the right nutrition for growth but they do get more wind, the bowel movements are more acid and it is easier to give them too much – overfeeding. There is no way of regulating what a bottle-fed baby takes in in the way that the breast does naturally. Bottle-fed babies need extra fluid too.

Health

Bottled milk does not contain the antibodies to protect the baby against infection and allergy that breast milk has. Babies can be safely bottle-fed, but great care is needed in keeping the bottles clean and free from infection.

Love

Bottle-fed babies need this just as much as breast-fed ones, but it may be tempting just to give the bottle. Touching and cuddling are very important to help the baby feel secure. **It is extremely dangerous to prop the bottle up with the baby on a cushion or in the cot.**

Cleaning and Sterilising Bottles

- ◆ Bottles should be washed in washing-up liquid, using a bottle brush to clean inside, then rinsed out under running water.
- ◆ The teats should be rinsed under running water.
- ◆ Bottles, teats and cleaning equipment (brushes) should be sterilised either by boiling for 20 minutes, or by using sterilising solution. The manufacturer's instructions should be followed carefully.

The Milk

It's best to stick to the same make and type of milk, whichever you choose. Follow the instructions on the packet carefully, stick to the amounts shown and only use the scoop provided in the packet. A day's feeds can be made up in one go and kept in the fridge.

The midwife and health visitor have a lot of experience of feeding problems and will advise on any difficulties.

Returning to 'Normal' in Body, Mind and Spirit after a Birth

After Pains

The uterus contracts rapidly after birth and many mothers are surprised to find a 'flat tummy' almost immediately afterwards. There is usually a feeling of relief about this. The uterus will continue to contract over the first three or four days until it is back to its pre-pregnancy size. These contractions are usually a little painful – the degree of pain seems to vary from mother to mother and from birth to birth. Breastfeeding, of course, stimulates the contractions and so there may be a stitch-like pain in the tummy when the baby is put to the breast. The pains don't usually last more than a few minutes, but if they are persistent, then a tablet or two of Paracetamol may bring some relief. Paracetamol does get into the breast milk, but there is no evidence of any harm coming to the baby from this. Try to look at these pains positively if possible, as part of the process of your body returning to normal after pregnancy and birth. Many other changes will be taking place. The pregnancy and the birth have used up some energy and mothers need to take some positive steps to regain physical fitness. Nutrition and exercise are the two areas of our lives over which we have some control, so these need attention just as they did in preparing for pregnancy (see Chapter One).

Bleeding and discharge

This is usual after the birth and for six to eight weeks afterwards. It shouldn't be heavy: no more, and usually rather less, than a period. If there is heavy bleeding, you should certainly tell your midwife or doctor. An offensive or smelly discharge may be a sign of infection, especially if the mother has a temperature too.

Healing tears, stitches, episiotomies and the perineum

This area can be sore for three or four days after the birth even without the added trauma of a tear or episiotomy. Warm baths help to relieve the soreness. We would recommend a few drops of homoeopathic calendula tincture in the bath to promote healing. We find that small tears heal better without stitching, but we don't have any research evidence for this.

TEARS AND EPISIOTOMIES

Evidence *Larger* tears and episiotomies do need stitches and the best and most comfortable way to do this is by *subcuticular* stitches – that is, underneath the skin, using absorbable materials; they don't need to be taken out, but dissolve themselves.

Stitched or not, the damage usually heals quickly. Some mothers experience bruising and swelling of the perineum. This can look very alarming but always resolves itself within a week or so. The discomfort can be relieved and the swelling reduced by cold applications with ice and by ultrasound administered by a physiotherapist. Homoeopathic Arnica, preferably in high potency (10M), taken as a single dose as soon as possible after the birth or after the damage appears, may also help. If bruising or soreness persists for three days or more after the birth, then Bellis Perennis 30c taken daily will help to heal the muscles and tissues.

Life will never be the same again so there are also psychological and spiritual changes to adjust to after a birth. Many people, with or without any religious experience or conviction, find the time immediately after the birth of a new baby very special. Some would describe it as 'holy'. It is certainly a time when mother, father and baby need to be together without disturbance for as long as possible and many new families value a quietness then. In hospital, this should be possible despite all the business going on around. At home, it should be easy to achieve. It will help to plan for this time immediately after the birth because it can be very easy to get wrapped up in giving news to the family, receiving visitors and organising life for the next few weeks, months and years. This time can be precious and shouldn't be missed, so try to plan for some peace and quiet for yourselves. Give visitors clear instructions about when to come and when to go. Leave the phone off the hook or on an answerphone, if possible. There will be plenty of time to give friends the good news and anyone with any sensitivity should understand your needs.

A Good Case History

Thomas, the author's middle son, born four days before Christmas, brought us the best and most peaceful Christmas ever. Family, for whom we always catered at Christmas, considerately stayed away. We had three days of peace, venturing out on Christmas Eve to church, to the surprise of our friends. Those few days gave us time to adjust and to prepare for the hard work of looking after the new baby.

Feeling High

Many mothers feel elated in the first few days after birth and who can blame them? What could be more exciting than giving birth and being with a new baby? Sometimes this excitement is such that it is difficult to sleep for the first night or even two. This is natural, but in hospital it may be attributed to being in a strange environment. Sleeping pills may be offered. Although the mother's desperation at being unable to sleep is understandable, we can't recommend the use of sleeping pills for the following reasons:

– the drugs get into the breast milk, and therefore into the baby;
– they will affect the mother's ability to wake in the night when the baby cries for a feed;
– the effects persist into the following day;
– the drugs used are nearly all addictive and addiction develops after as little as a week of use.

Homoeopathic coffea 30c is safer. Or Kali phos 30c may help if you are mentally exhausted, suffering from a headache and, despite feeling tired, are too excited to sleep.

The 'Blues'

After the high, there may well be a low. The 'baby blues', in fact, affect 50 to 70 per cent of mothers. It happens between the fourth and tenth days after birth and can be very distressing to mothers and their families especially if it is unexpected, so **be prepared** and prepare your family.

Some of the things mothers may experience are disturbed sleep, perhaps with vivid or frightening dreams. On waking, there may be a short time when you are unsure where you are or what you are doing. Some mothers may experience hallucinations on waking. The main feeling is one of emotional over-reactivity. Moods fluctuate from happy and laughing to floods of tears. Small problems seem to be enormous ones and can provoke strong reactions.

Mothers often feel very anxious at this time. This anxiety is often associated with problems to do with breastfeeding, especially as this coincides with the time when the milk comes in and there may be problems with engorgement. There may be feelings of hostility, often directed at partners, but also sometimes at midwives, though rarely at the baby. Midwives are used to this, but husbands or partners need to be prepared. The blues rarely lasts more than two or three days and does not require any medical treatment, merely understanding and sympathy from the mother's supporters. Because of its timing, it is often explained as being due to changes in hormone levels, but there is no evidence for this. Low potency homoeopathic Pulsatilla may help. Mothers may need extra rest and sleep at this time. If Dad can help to give her a quiet hour or two free from the new baby's demands, this will be a welcome break and will help in emotional healing, as well as with the father's bonding to the baby.

Postnatal Depression (PND)

Between 10 and 20 per cent of mothers are affected by postnatal depression which can occur at any time after the birth, up to the end of the first year. Childbirth is generally regarded as a 'happy event', but for mothers experiencing 'PND', life for themselves and their families can be miserable. Furthermore, the research evidence shows that postnatal depression has serious consequences not only for the mother, but also for the baby. It may also trigger other mental health problems and can be a disrupting factor in a marriage.

Unrecognised misery

Research shows that PND is often unrecognised by the mother herself, her family and health professionals. Recently, however, there has been growing awareness of the problem, especially by health visitors and midwives who are trained to be on the lookout for symptoms. There may be many reasons why the problem is hidden below the surface. Perhaps 'the blues' described above, being accepted as a normal consequence of birth, means that a mother who remains depressed for longer is accepted by her family as being normal. Birth is expected to be 'happy' and mothers may conceal their true feelings in order to comply with what their family and society expect of them. Health professionals may still be slow to recognise the condition.

The Symptoms of Postnatal Depression

- **Low Mood** Feeling sad and gloomy most of the time. Tearfulness and feelings of hopelessness or despair. Some mothers have suicidal thoughts but usually suppress these 'for the sake of the baby'. Mothers feel very emotional and react strongly to situations they would usually take in their stride. Television programmes, especially about natural disasters, may cause intense emotion. This low mood may be variable from day to day.
- **Anxiety** Worries about minor problems, the baby, money. Depressed mothers may be unable to tolerate the baby crying. Often it is very difficult to share the worries with family or friends for fear of over-burdening them. This may result in a feeling of isolation and increasing irritability with family, especially the husband or partner.
- **Poor Sleep** Of course sleep is likely to be disturbed by the baby anyway, but depressed mothers often wake in the night, typically between two and three in the morning, and can't get back to sleep. They feel tired despite a good night. Sometimes depression causes too much sleep – wanting to sleep during the day, and still not feeling refreshed.
- **Lack of Energy** Everything is 'too much trouble'. There's a feeling of 'I can't be bothered'. Some depressed mothers say that they know what they have to do to look after the baby or the household, but their arms and legs just won't let them do it.
- **Poor Appetite** No interest or enjoyment of food for themselves, though often mothers have to keep cooking for the family.

- ◆ **Inability to Cope** This can be the most distressing feeling for someone who before being pregnant was busy, energetic and capable. It can be difficult to make even the most ordinary day-to-day decisions such as what to wear. The result is loss of self-esteem and guilt about being ineffective as a wife and mother.
- ◆ **Poor Concentration and Memory** This can also be very distressing because of the feeling of being out of control – 'What ever is happening to me?'.

In addition to the above, loss of libido or interest in sex is a feature of depression which may be normal during the first year after a birth. There may be physical difficulties because of damage to the perineum, stitches or healing tears as well as psychological difficulties.

Recognising Postnatal Depression

If you are a mother in the first year after the birth of a baby, and some of the descriptions above seem to apply to you, then you may be suffering from depression. Seek help soon, because there is effective treatment. If you are still unsure about whether you are suffering from this condition, then go through the questionnaire in Chapter One. If you score more than 12 points, you are probably suffering from postnatal depression.

Treatment of Postnatal Depression

Family doctors are experts in treating depression because it is a condition most of them meet every week. Only if a mother has a complex problem, possibly requiring hospital admission, should it be necessary for referral to a psychiatrist. Most doctors will adopt a two-pronged approach to treating depression. The two arms of treatment are:

- listening and supporting – which may be undertaken by a trained counsellor or psychologist, or by a midwife or health visitor with suitable training;
- pharmaceutical treatment with antidepressants. These are of two main types – tricyclics such as imipramine, amitryptiline or dothiepin, and the newer 'SSRIs' such as fluoxetene (Prozac) and paroxetene.

ANTIDEPRESSANTS

Evidence shows the undoubted efficacy of these drugs in the treatment of depression. They can, if used appropriately, help to transform lives from misery to normality.

The disadvantages, as with all effective medicine, are the side effects. The tricyclics can cause a dry mouth (which is the most common complaint), constipation, dizziness and, rarely but seriously, cardiac arrhythmias (irregular heart rhythm). Some are sedative and may cause a feeling of being 'doped'. The SSRIs have a long list of possible side effects but are considered to be less 'toxic' than the older tricyclics. They have the disadvantage of a withdrawal syndrome when they are stopped, but this does not affect everyone. In rare cases, they can also cause a syndrome rather like Parkinson's disease, but this is reversible when the drug is stopped. Many of these side effects wear off after a week or two of taking the tablets.

Another disadvantage of all antidepressants is that there is not an immediate improvement in mood. The effect takes ten days to two weeks to come on. If you are someone who has been prescribed one of these drugs, it is important to keep taking it each day even though at first you may notice no improvement in your mood. Eventually the medicine will work. The dose may need adjusting too; often treatment is abandoned either by the doctor or the patient because of lack of effect, when an increase to an appropriate dose might have produced a good result.

Some health districts have set up specialist services for postnatal mental health problems. Often they are in the form of a 'drop-in' clinic where no referral is required. The health visitor will know about these, but information can also be found from local branches of MIND.

Prevention of Postnatal Depression

Once having experienced postnatal depression, unfortunately the risk is increased for the same woman in a subsequent pregnancy. The risk of PND is 60 to 75 per cent if it has occurred previously. There is some evidence to suggest that it can be prevented, reducing the risk to about 50 per cent by treatment during the pregnancy. It doesn't seem to matter whether the treatment is by support and counselling, or by drugs. There are some doctors who enthusiastically promote the hormone progesterone given immediately after the birth as a preventive measure, but the evidence for this treatment is not convincing.

Caroline suffered from PND after her first pregnancy. The experience was so dreadful that she was extremely frightened when she became pregnant again four years later. She had needed referral to the psychiatric service, and for the second pregnancy we liaised with her psychiatrist and gave her a programme that we hoped would help to prevent a recurrence of her depression. We used hypnosis throughout the pregnancy to help her manage her anxiety. We gave her supportive counselling. In the last two months she took a tricycle antidepressant and, for good measure, since she had read about progesterone and wished to try it, we gave her injections after the birth. She had no recurrence of her depression. Which treatment was the effective one? We still don't know, but for Caroline, her husband and first son, there was immense relief.

The Postnatal Check-up

There is now a tradition of going to the doctor's, or sometimes to the hospital, six weeks after the birth, for a 'check-up'. Family doctors encourage this because they receive a fee for it from the health authority. It seems to us that there is actually little purpose in this check-up and it seems to have passed into folklore as a ritual in the same way that women used to go to church after the birth of a baby. Many doctors now try to make the visit more useful to mothers, and more efficient, by giving the baby a check-up at the same time, and giving the first vaccinations.

We adopt this approach and, in addition, try to give the mother space to tell us of any problems or concerns. It is also traditional to have a cervical smear at the 'postnatal', and a vaginal examination. Some doctors are questioning the value of the smear as the results may not be reliable because of the changes in the cervix remaining after the birth. Most would agree that the vaginal examination is unnecessary and intrusive. Research is needed to re-evaluate the postnatal check-up, but our advice to mothers is to use it positively. Go armed with a list of questions. Take the baby because the six week check-up is certainly useful for he or she. It may also be a good time to discuss contraception.

And Now?

The birth and the baby are just the beginning. Perhaps we should all keep this in perspective. Families experience much joy together as well as some pain. Who can tell what the future will hold for mother, father and baby? Eventually, the baby may have babies of his or her own.

GLOSSARY

....

Alpha-fetoprotein (AFP) A protein that is made by all developing babies, which is found in the mother's blood. It is used as a marker for Downs' syndrome (lower than average levels) and for spina bifida (higher levels).

Amniocentesis A test for chromosome abnormalities that is done by taking a small amount of the fluid around the baby by putting a needle through the mother's tummy into the uterus. The fetal cells in the fluid are analysed to check the chromosomes.

Apgar Score Points out of ten for the baby's condition at birth based on colour, breathing, muscle tone, reflexes and heart rate. It provides a quick, but crude, way of assessing whether a baby needs to have special care.

Breech The baby's bottom, and sometimes the feet, present first to the outside world.

Brow Presentation The baby's forehead presents to the cervix instead of the back of the head. This makes delivery very difficult. Sometimes a caesarean section may be needed.

Cephalic The baby's head presents first to the outside world.

Cervix The neck of the womb. It must open first to allow the baby to be born.

Chloasma Dark skin on the face in pregnancy; thought to be caused by hormone changes.

Chromosome Microscopic threads contained in every cell of the body, which carry the genes, the 'blueprint' for a living being.

Crowning When the widest part of the baby's head passes through the vaginal opening as it is born.

CVS (Chorionic Villus Sampling) A means of diagnosing chromosome abnormalities (similar to amniocentesis). A needle is inserted into the uterus, through which a sample of the early placental tissue is removed. This can then be checked for the baby's chromosomes.

Downs' syndrome The baby has an extra chromosome 23. Downs' babies have certain facial characteristics and are usually slow to develop and below average intelligence. They may also have heart problems.

EDD Estimated Date of Delivery, calculated from the date of the last menstrual period.

Embryo The baby during the first 12 weeks in the womb.

Engagement If the widest part of the baby's head has passed through the opening into the pelvis, it is said to be 'engaged'.

Episiotomy A cut made through the perineum from the opening of the vagina to allow more room for the baby's head to be born.

Fallopian Tubes The two tubes connecting the uterus to the ovaries. An egg passes through the fallopian tube on one side each month after ovulation.

Fetus The unborn baby.

Fetal Distress If, during labour, the baby is not receiving enough oxygen, there is said to be 'fetal distress'. There are signs of fetal distress which midwives and doctors recognise.

Fontanelle The 'soft spot' on top of the baby's head.

Fundus The top of the uterus.

Gestation The length of time since conception.

Hypertension High blood pressure.

Liquor The fluid around the baby in the womb.

LMP Last Menstrual Period.

Malpresentation Means that part of the baby is 'presenting' to the cervix which may cause difficulty in the birth. For example, a brow presentation, where the baby's forehead is the presenting part, may cause a very difficult labour requiring caesarean section if the malpresentation cannot be corrected.

Meconium The black tarry motions passed by all babies when they first have their bowels open. If found in the liquor during labour, meconium may be a sign of fetal distress.

Moulding The flexible changes in the shape of a baby's head as it passes through the birth canal.

Obstetrician A doctor who specialises in the care of pregnant women.

Oedema Swelling in the fingers, hands or ankles due to fluid retention.

Oestriol A kind of oestrogen.

Oestrogen A hormone produced by the ovaries and in pregnancy by the placenta.

Oligohydramnios Too little fluid surrounding the baby in the womb. May be associated with kidney problems in the baby.

Pelvic Floor The skin, muscles and ligaments in the perineum which support the organs in the pelvis.

Perineum The part of the body between the anus and the vagina.

Placenta The afterbirth, a large, flat organ which joins the baby to the mother by attaching to the wall of the womb. The umbilical cord joins the baby to the placenta.

Placenta Praevia The placenta lies either partly or wholly over the cervix. If it wholly covers the cervix, birth will be obstructed and caesarean section is necessary.

Polyhydramnios Excessive fluid around the baby in the womb. It can be associated with pre-eclampsia or with premature labour or malpresentations. Also with abnormalities of the baby's head or oesophagus.

Pre-eclampsia A serious condition affecting a small number of women in the last two months of pregnancy. High blood pressure, protein in the urine and oedema are the signs.

Progesterone The hormone produced by the placenta in large amounts during pregnancy.

Puerperium The time immediately after childbirth during which the mother recovers. It lasts about six weeks.

Quickening The baby's first movements felt by the mother.

Rubella German measles which, if contracted in early pregnancy, can result in abnormalities for the baby.

Spina Bifida The baby's spine and spinal cord fail to close over properly. The severity varies. Surgery can correct most cases, but severe cases cause paralysis.

TENS (Transcutaneous electrical nerve stimulation) A method of pain relief which works by producing tiny electrical currents from a device which is attached to the body. It can be used in labour.

Transverse Lie The baby is lying across the mother's abdomen in the uterus. From this position, vaginal birth is impossible. Either the lie must change or a caesarean section would be required for birth.

Trimester A three-month period in pregnancy.

Umbilicus Naval or tummy button.

Vernix The creamy substance which covers some babies at birth. It is perfectly normal.

Vertex The top part of the baby's head.

ADDRESSES

....

Active Birth Centre
55 Dartmouth Park Road
London NW5 1SL
(0171 627 3006)

AIMS (Association for Improvement in Maternity Services)
40 Kingswood Avenue
London NW6 6LS
(0181 960 5585)

Association for Postnatal Illness
25 Jerdan Place
London SW6 1BE
(0171 386 0868 10am–5pm)

Association of Breastfeeding Mothers
26 Holmshaw Close
London SE26 4TG
(*24-hour service* 0181 778 4769)

British Acupuncture Association and Registrar
34 Alderney Street
London SW1V 4EU
(0171 834 1012)

British Homoeopathic Association
27a Devonshire Street
London W1N 1RJ
(0171 935 2163)

British Reflexology Association
Monks Orchard
Whitbourne
Worcester
WR6 5RB

Centre for Pregnancy Nutrition
University of Sheffield
(*Eating for pregnancy 24-hour helpline* 0114 242 4084)

Family Rights Group
18 Ashwin Street
London E8 3DL
(0171 249 0008)
Advice on statutory rights Mon–Fri 1.30–3pm

FORESIGHT
28 The Paddock
Godalming
Surrey GU7 1XD
(01483) 427839

Independent Midwives Association
94 Auckland Road
London
SE19 2DB

La Leche League
BCM 3424
London WC1N 3XX
(0171 242 1278)

MAMA (Meet a Mum Association)
3 Woodside Avenue
London SE25
Offers moral support and practical help to women suffering from postnatal depression. Support is available through local groups or from mothers who have experienced the problem. Write for information on local groups enclosing a stamped addressed envelope.

Maternity Alliance
15 Britannia Street
London WC1X 9JP
(0171 837 1265)
Advice on maternity care and state benefits

MIND
Granta House
15-19 Broadway
Stratford
London E15 4BQ
(0181 519 2122)

Miscarriage Association
Clayton Hospital
Northgate
Wakefield
West Yorkshire
WF1 3JS
(01924 200799)

National Association for Maternal and Child Welfare
40-42 Osnaburgh Street
London NW1 3ND
(0171 383 4115/4117/4541)
Counselling

NCT (National Childbirth Trust)
Alexandra House
Oldham Terrace
Acton
London W3 6NH
(0181 992 8637)
Support in pregnancy and breast-feeding

The Society of Homoeopaths
2 Artizan Road
Northampton NN1 4HU
(01604 21400)

TAMBA (Twins and Multiple Births Association)
PO Box 30
Little Sutton
South Wirral L66 1TH
(0151 3348 0020)

INDEX